Comments on **Heart Health – the '**
guide *from reade*

'Your book has given me more support than any doctor, hospital or support group. I found it very informative and it answered a lot of questions I forgot to ask when talking to the doctor.'

Gwyneth Fenton, London

'I found great comfort and an insight into my illness after reading this book.'

D. Bradley, Falkirk

'Of the books we have consulted, we have found yours the more accessible and helpful.'

V Butters, Coventry

'I always keep the book to hand and I always dip into it when I want to know something. The book is well written, and very straightforward and understandable and I will gladly recommend this book to anyone who has a heart problem.'

Ian Golding, Darlington

Reviews of Heart Health – the 'at your fingertips' guide

'Busy doctors, or dissatisfied heart patients, couldn't do better than invest in Dr Jackson's latest book Heart health at your fingertips. It contains 260 pages devoted to questions that patients ask and answers the doctor wishes he had given if only he'd had the time to think how best to put them.'

Dr Thomas Stuttaford, *The Times*

'Those readers who want to know more about the various treatments for heart disease will be much enlightened.'

Dr James Le Fanu, *Daily Telegraph*

'One of the most straightforward and helpful books on heart disease that I have ever read . . . Dr Jackson isn't lecturing me, but rather he is sitting alongside me, answering my questions in a way that makes sense to me.'

Heart News

'Visits to the surgery or the hospital are often not the best time or setting for patients to receive answers to questions or concerns. Those who have experienced this frustration will find Dr Jackson's book a most useful and informative resource. Heart health at your fingertips comes highly recommended.'

The Family Heart Digest

'Here's a book you might want to have to hand for all those questions you would like to ask but don't know where or who to consult. Dr Jackson gives straightforward advice together with all the latest information about coronary heart disease.'

In Balance magazine

'The medical expertise of Consultant Cardiologist Dr Graham Jackson is now available to people all over the UK.'

People, Guy's & St Thomas' Hospitals magazine

'The joy of this book is that it is not a medical textbook but a book giving information about the practical problems of heart disease and its prevention or treatment. It is easy reading, dip in and out, with a format of questions and answers – questions we all want to ask followed by well thought out answers. Highly recommended.'

Heart Digest

'I would recommend this book to any patient or member of the general public expressing an interest in keeping their heart health.'

British Journal of Cardiology

'I found the book easy to read, and would recommend it, especially in today's climate with the national emphasis on coronary heart disease.'

The Pharmaceutical Journal

At Your Fingertips

HEART HEALTH

THIRD EDITION

Graham Jackson FESC, FACC, FRCP
*Consultant Cardiologist, Guys and St Thomas' Hospital Trust,
St Thomas' Hospital, London SE1*

CLASS PUBLISHING • LONDON

Text © Graham Jackson 2000
© Class Publishing (London) Ltd 2000

Printing history
First published 1998
Second edition 2000
Reprinted 2000
Reprinted with revisions 2000
Third edition 2004

The authors and publishers welcome feedback from the users of this book. Please contact the publishers.

Class Publishing (London) Ltd, Barb House, Barb Mews, London W6 7PA, UK
Telephone: 020 7371 2119
[International +4420]
Fax: 020 7371 2878
Email: post@class.co.uk
Visit our website – www.class.co.uk

A CIP catalogue record for this book is available from the British Library

ISBN 1 85959 097 7

Edited by Michèle Clarke

Cartoons by Linda Moore

Illustrations by David Woodroffe

Indexed by Val Elliston

Designed by Wendy Bann

Typesetting by Martin Bristow

Printed and bound in Finland by WS Bookwell, Juva

Contents

Acknowledgements   xi

Foreword by *Professor Brian L Pentecost* MD FRCP   xiii

Foreword to the Third Edition by *Dr Graham Jackson*   xv

INTRODUCTION   xvii
   How to use this book   xix
   Questions for your doctor or practice nurse   xx
   Finally   xx

CHAPTER 1 *How your heart works*   1
   Anatomy of the heart   2
   How your heart works   7
   What can go wrong with my heart?   9

CHAPTER 2 *Coronary artery disease*   11
   Risks of smoking   13
   Risks of high blood pressure   27
   Risks of high cholesterol levels   48
   Other risk factors for coronary heart disease   61
   Women and coronary heart disease   67

CHAPTER 3 *Angina*   75
   Symptoms   76
   Tests   81
   Treatment   91
   Other treatments for angina   125

CHAPTER 4 *Heart attacks*   132
  Symptoms   134
  Heart attack – the event   137
  Recovery period   142
  Emotional problems after a heart attack   145
  Treatment   147
  Helping yourself   150

CHAPTER 5 *Heart failure*   157
  Causes   158
  Symptoms   160
  Tests   163
  Treatment   167

CHAPTER 6 *Palpitations*   178
  Types of palpitations   179
  Self-help   182
  Tests   185
  Treatment   187
  Atrial fibrillation   189
  Other abnormal heart beats   196
  Blackouts   201

CHAPTER 7 *Valve disease*   203
  Causes   204
  Symptoms   205
  Tests   205
  Treatment   206
  Infection   209

CHAPTER 8 *Sex and the heart*   211
  Questions that you may feel are difficult to ask
     your doctor!   212

CHAPTER 9 *Diet*   225
  Food types and eating healthily   226
  Losing weight   249

CHAPTER 10 *Exercise*   264
   Why bother?   264
   How much?   270
   Safety   271
   Choosing your exercise   272

GLOSSARY   280

APPENDIX 1 *Practising what I preach!*   288

APPENDIX 2 *Useful addresses*   291

APPENDIX 3 *Useful publications*   300

APPENDIX 4 *Height to weight – adults (desirable)*   302

INDEX   304

LIFESTYLE HINTS

	page numbers
Complementary medicine	125–30
Depression	147
Diabetes	65–6
Driving	112, 123, 198
Exercising	264–79
Gardening	122
Healthy eating	232–3
HRT	68–74
Illegal drugs	66–7
Losing weight	249–51
Sex and relationships	211–24
Stopping smoking	18–21
Stress reduction	62–3
Travel and holidays	123–4, 161–2, 198

Dedication

For Maggie, Keira and Matthew

Acknowledgements

It would have been impossible to write this book without the help of Michèle Clarke and Richard Warner. To Michèle, my especial thanks for helping me write plain English and being supportive when it all seemed overwhelming. I am grateful to Professor Brian Pentecost for providing such a warm foreword and checking the text for clarity and mistakes. Dr Richard Wray, Dr Ian Baird and Professor John Swales reviewed the text and provided extremely helpful suggestions and identified areas that I had not made clear or helpful. Azmina Govinda with her expert knowledge as a consultant nutritionist has made sure that the sections on diet and lifestyle make sense. I would like to thank Linda Moore for the delightful cartoons, David Woodroffe for the clear illustrations and Wendy Bann for the overall design. I must also thank Geoffrey Segrove and his charming family for agreeing to appear on the front cover and finally I need to acknowledge all my patients who have gladly provided most of the questions and have in turn helped me answer them I hope in a way that is helpful and clear.

Foreword

by Professor Brian L Pentecost MD FRCP
Former Medical Director of the British Heart Foundation

When we are happy and feeling well, it is only natural to put aside all thoughts of illness. Life, after all, is meant to be enjoyed. Many people are, however, aware that heart disease, particularly coronary artery disease, can brutally interrupt that happiness. In the UK and many other parts of the developed world, death from heart attacks and other complications of coronary artery disease, reached its peak in the late 1970s and is now slowly in decline. Unhappily, coronary artery disease remains the single most important cause of premature death in this country. Death from heart disease is not always as quick and painless as is sometimes thought. Many people suffer a prolonged period of disability as the result of chest pain and breathlessness. Yet, to a large extent, coronary artery disease is preventable, not completely of course, but we can certainly improve our chances of avoiding heart disease by quite simple manoeuvres. It is often said that the advice on preventing heart disease is confused and conflicting, particularly over the matter of what is 'healthy eating'. This is really not true, as Dr Graham Jackson makes abundantly clear in this book. There will always be some debate over details, but the broad thrust of dietary advice, particularly concerning a reduction in animal fats and an increase in fresh fruit and vegetables, finds favour with the vast majority of experts in the field. So, too, does the advice about regular physical activity and avoiding cigarette smoking. Graham Jackson illustrates very well the fact that reducing the risks of heart disease does not require complicated dietary regimens or joining expensive health clubs.

Some readers will already have symptoms of coronary heart disease. For those, the new world of tests and possible treatments can be totally bewildering. The language and terminology alone is enough to terrify you! Graham Jackson takes the reader on a voyage of discovery and explanation in his clearly written and good humoured text, which should allay fear through awareness of what heart disease is all about.

Foreword to the Third Edition

Sometimes medical advice seems contradictory – one minute it's one recommendation and the next it is another. That is the nature of research and progress. A series of events may come together to lead to the belief that a form of diet or treatment will be of benefit but that belief must be translated into proof. Sometimes what appear to be good ideas just do not work when rigorously tested. This third edition therefore contains changes that reflect new knowledge about the heart and how to not only treat the conditions that can affect the heart but also help prevent heart disease. We do not have all the answers to every question, but in this book I will attempt to answer as many as possible. Once more to the many people who have written to me – thank you for your comments and suggestions.

Introduction

This book is principally about your heart: how to keep it strong or, if it has been weakened in some way, how to make it as strong as possible. The major cause of weakening of your heart is called coronary artery disease (CAD). The coronary arteries are those arteries which feed the heart itself. They arise from the main artery leaving the heart, the aorta, and run around the outside of the heart, sending many branches into the heart's muscle. They deliver oxygen and energy so that the heart can do its job of pumping blood around the body. If the coronary arteries become narrowed, the blood supply to the heart will be restricted. The result is that when the heart needs to beat faster (e.g. when you are walking up a hill), your heart will be starved of energy and begin to complain, usually by causing chest pain (known as angina). If a coronary artery blocks completely, there will a sudden loss of blood to a portion of heart muscle, chemicals build up, you will experience severe pain and a heart attack occurs as the muscle stops working . If a big coronary artery blocks, the heart attack will be large, but if a small artery is blocked, only a small loss of muscle will happen.

Coronary disease is our greatest medical enemy and as much a threat to women as to men. Women may think of it as a man's disease, but it is an equal opportunity killer with no respect for sex, race or religion. Coronary heart disease kills nearly 170 000 men and women in the UK each year, and in America 500 000 adults die each year of coronary artery disease; half of these are women. This means that an average of 460 people a day (or one person every three minutes) die from coronary artery disease in the UK. Women may be more afraid of breast cancer but it is five times as likely that they will die from the consequences of heart disease. It is so common that one in three adults of both sexes over 65 years of age has some form of heart disease.

The cost of coronary disease affects both you personally (causing stress and uncertainty, and affecting social and family life) and the community, with a National Health Service bill for heart disease per year estimated to be over 3500 million pounds. The key to preventing coronary disease happening *to you* is to understand the causes and to know how to reduce the chances of it developing. It is *never* too late to act for yourself and your family.

In this book you will discover how the heart works and how coronary artery disease develops. Prevention is emphasized. Prevention before heart problems occur is called primary prevention, and prevention after you have been diagnosed as having coronary disease is called secondary prevention. Both are important – when you have a disease, you want to stop it getting worse, and when you have no evidence of disease, you want to keep it that way. Sections of this book are concerned with diet, exercise, smoking and blood pressure control, and the importance of reducing your risk factors for coronary disease. A risk factor is something that increases your likelihood of developing a disease, and an easy example of this is cigarette smoking. Smokers have more coronary disease than non-smokers, and smokers who quit reduce their risk to the same as non-smokers after a period of 4–5 years. Advice is given on risk factors and how to minimize your risk.

The consequences of coronary artery disease are discussed with advice on treatments available, and how you can help yourself. Doctors need to have good evidence that a form of treatment is effective and this is known as 'evidence-based medicine'. It is important that you understand the benefits and risks of any therapy recommended to you: be fully informed and ask questions – it's your heart after all! Just as I must provide evidence that medical treatments are effective, you must ask for similar evidence from unconventional treatments that you may have read about: do not believe all you are told – ask for the evidence. Remember, however, that evidence is of a very varied quality. It is easy to be convinced on the basis of personal or a close friend's or relative's experience that the disease has been 'cured'. It is unfortunately easy to be deluded as most diseases are very variable and impressions of a 'cure' may be misguided. The only way to establish genuine benefit is from scientific trials. These try to remove chance or, put another way, remove the possibility that you would have got better anyway.

Sections on angina, heart attacks, drugs and bypass surgery, and the role of angioplasty (balloon treatment) and stent placement (an expandable metal cage) to hold arteries open, is covered in detail.

This is not a medical textbook but a book giving information about the practical problems of coronary artery disease and its prevention or treatment. It deals with the commonest questions asked and tries to answer in the clearest way. Not all questions have easy answers so, where there are grey areas, these are discussed in an attempt to clarify what, for doctors as well as patients, can be a difficult subject.

Coronary artery disease can be thought of as a series of keys – the first key is the key to prevention, the second the key to early recognition of warning symptoms, the third the key to the correct treatment, and the fourth the key to preventing it happening again. This book is about finding the keys and information is vital for finding these keys. Armed with this book, you will be in a good position to find these keys.

How to use this book

If you do not understand the terms used, check in the glossary at the back. The book is written in a way that allows you to dip into it, rather than read it from cover to cover. It's a good idea to read Chapter 1 before any other, just to be sure that you understand how the heart works. With a good background, the rest is easier to follow.

You may want to know about drug treatment for angina (see the section on **Treatment** in Chapter 3) but it's best to see how it compares with other treatments in order to get a broader view and to see what options are available. The same applies to heart attack patients or their relatives – read around the subject to get a better perspective.

Questions for your doctor or practice nurse

Books like this try to answer as many questions as possible, but they should encourage you to ask your doctor questions also. No one ever remembers to ask questions in the surgery. Write your questions down before you visit the surgery, making a list like a shopping list. If your doctor cannot answer them, write to me (at the publisher's address at the beginning of this book) and I shall try to answer them for you.

Finally

- Don't be afraid of heart disease.
- Learn about it to understand it.
- Do your best to prevent it.
- Learn to cope with it; and
- Remember, despite suffering heart problems, most people lead full and active lives as a result of modern treatments.

1
How your heart works

Your heart is a muscle pump which pushes blood through your arteries to all organs of your body. The body needs oxygen and energy to work normally and blood is the delivery system. Blood picks up its oxygen in the lungs and becomes bright red as a result. After it gives up its oxygen, blood takes carbon dioxide and waste products for elimination to the lungs, liver and kidneys in the veins, where it is a now a dark red colour. Your heart muscle needs oxygen and energy and this is obtained from the blood through the coronary arteries. Disease of the coronary arteries is the commonest cause of death and disability in the western world because it stops the heart – the body's engine – doing its job properly.

Anatomy of the heart

What is the heart?

The heart is a muscle pump but it is a very sophisticated one. It is made of muscle different from the sort that moves your arms and legs. Heart muscle is particularly strong as it has to cope with the physical and emotional stresses of normal daily life and, of course, it never takes a rest (you hope!). It beats on average 100 000 times every 24 hours and pumps out between 5 and 20 litres of blood (1 litre equals just under 2 pints) every minute depending on your body's needs – more when you are being active than when you are resting. Every organ in the body needs oxygen to function normally and efficiently.

Fresh blood in the arteries delivers oxygen and energy to your body tissues and then, when it has given up its energy supply, blood carries away in the veins unwanted waste products including carbon dioxide. The heart is the engine that pumps the blood around; normally it is the size of a clenched fist.

Can you tell me what the coronary arteries are?

These are the tubes or vessels that supply your heart muscle with the oxygen and energy that it needs to pump efficiently. The vessels that carry the oxygen round the body are called *arteries*. Coronary arteries* are tough tubes able to cope with the pressure pumped out by the heart. They are often confused with *veins*, such as those that we see on the back of the hand or on the legs (usually blue). Veins bring used-up blood back to the heart. They

* There is a glossary at the back of the book to help you with unfamiliar terms.

are thinner than arteries and do not work or cope with high pressure in the same way as arteries do.

There are three important coronary arteries with many branches. There is a left coronary artery which divides into two large branches, and a right coronary artery which is usually one big vessel (Figure 1.1). The coronary arteries arise from the main artery leaving your heart (the *aorta*), beginning just above the aortic valve (see question below). The most important coronary

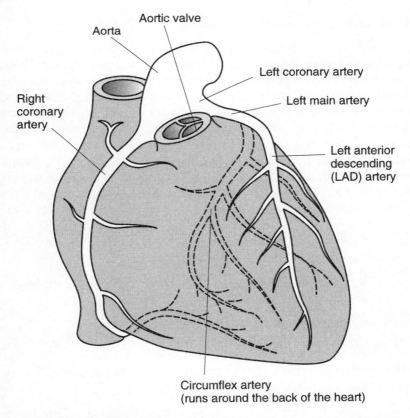

Figure 1.1 The coronary arteries surround the heart muscle and send branches into the muscle, delivering blood containing oxygen. They start from the aorta just above the aortic valve. Dotted lines indicate the arteries running around the back of the heart.

artery is the left main stem, which controls both branches of the left coronary artery and, as a result, most of the blood supply to your heart muscle. Think of your coronary arteries like the branches of a big tree with a main trunk branching out into smaller and smaller branches and twigs. The coronary arteries start at about 3–4 mm in size (like a thin straw) and as they feed the muscle they divide to reach all the layers of muscle. They run around the outside of the heart, sending their branches inwards.

What happens when things go wrong with the coronary arteries?

The inner lining of your arteries is called the endothelium (pronounced *en-doe-thee-li-um*) which is a smooth surface allowing the blood to flow easily. If the endothelium becomes damaged, the tube becomes narrower, and the blood flow becomes turbulent with a chance of clots forming. Think of the artery as a roadway with a new road surface (the endothelium) – now imagine what happens to traffic flow if pot holes are allowed to develop and road works cone off one or two lanes or humps are introduced – drive too fast and you will come a cropper! Your endothelium can become damaged by:

- cigarette smoking;
- poorly treated high blood pressure; and
- a high level of cholesterol in your blood, causing localized deposits of fatty material (road humps!).

Narrowed coronary arteries can cause:

- angina;
- heart attack (the medical term for this is *myocardial* (heart muscle) *infarction* (death) (see Chapter 3);
- irregular heart beats (some types of palpitations) (see Chapter 5); and heart failure (where your muscle becomes weak) (see Chapter 4).

What is the aorta?

The aorta is the main artery leaving your heart. It sends blood to your head and then curves over to run down your chest along the spine. It passes along the back of your stomach, and at the top of the legs it divides into the big arteries, which send branches down to your feet.

What are the valves?

The valves control the flow of blood into and out of your heart. They open and shut just like a tap being turned on and off. When working normally, they act as one-way valves. The valves are on the inside of your heart, whereas the coronary arteries are on the outside.

There are four valves – the aortic, mitral, pulmonary and tricuspid. Look at Figure 1.2 and see the sequence of events.

1. Blood returns to your heart through the veins. It has given up its oxygen to your brain, kidneys and muscle. It comes from the head region in a big vein called the *superior* (from the top of the body) *vena cava*, and from the lower body in a big vein called the *inferior vena cava*. It collects in a chamber called the right *atrium*.

2. The *tricuspid valve* separates this collecting chamber from the right ventricle, which is part of your muscle pump. (*Ventricle* is the medical word for pump.) You will notice the use of the word 'right' at this stage. This is because your heart is divided into two sides – the right, which collects used-up blood and passes it to your lungs to pick up oxygen, and the left, which collects oxygen-rich blood from the lungs and pumps it round the body. The muscle pump on the left is called the left ventricle. This is the most important part of the heart and the one that is most often damaged in a heart attack.

3. On the left side of your heart, blood leaving the lungs has been collecting in the left atrium. Blood therefore collects in

the right atrium and left atrium at the same time. Separating the left atrium from the left ventricle is the *mitral valve*. The mitral valve opens at the same time as the tricuspid valve so that blood enters the right and left ventricles simultaneously.

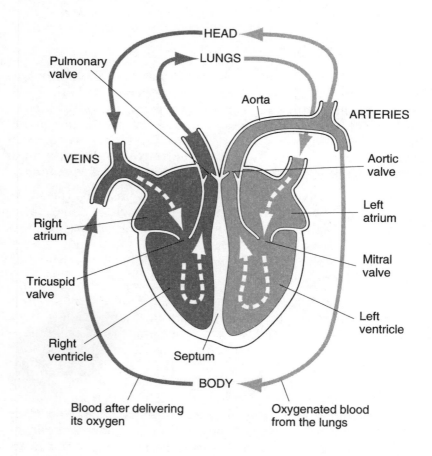

Figure 1.2 The circulation of blood from the body through the heart to the lungs. From the lungs the blood containing oxygen returns to the heart and circulates to the rest of the body. The atria are the collecting chambers; the ventricles are the muscle pump.

4. Both the right ventricle and left ventricle contract at the same time. As the pressure builds up, the force closes the tricuspid and mitral valves (preventing any leaking backwards) and opens the *pulmonary* and *aortic valves.* Blood is ejected through the pulmonary valve to your lungs, and the aortic valve to your body. When the pump has emptied, the pressure drops, the pulmonary and aortic valves close, and the tricuspid and mitral valves open again; the cycle is then repeated.

What keeps the right and left heart apart?

The muscle that divides your heart is called the *septum.* Between the right and left atrium, it is known as the atrial septum, and between the ventricles, the ventricular septum. When a hole occurs in your heart, we call it a defect – between the atria (plural of atrium), it is known as an *atrial septal defect* (ASD) and, between the ventricles, it is known as a *ventricular septal defect* (VSD).

How your heart works

When I asked my doctor how my heart works, he said that it would take too long to explain! Can you tell me simply how the normal heart works?

The healthy normal heart is made up of strong muscle and four valves in full working order. It gets its oxygen from the coronary arteries. It is controlled by an electric circuit which tells it when to beat and how fast to beat. The medical term for contraction of your heart pump (i. e. when the heart beats – felt as the pulse) is *systole,* and when the heart relaxes (between the beats or pulse), *diastole.*

The nurse at our practice runs a clinic to test blood pressures. What is blood pressure exactly and why is it so important?

We all need a blood pressure to keep our blood flowing round our bodies. It is the pressure of the blood in the arteries that is needed for delivering oxygen and food where it is needed and taking away waste products to the kidneys and liver.

Blood pressure has two terms applied to it – systolic and diastolic. The *systolic pressure* is the top pressure and is at its maximum following each heart beat. The bottom pressure (*diastolic pressure*) is the lowest recording between heart beats when your heart is resting. You might see, for example, 120 (systolic)/80 (diastolic) given as millimetres of mercury and, as mercury's symbol is Hg, you will see 120/80 mmHg, or for shorthand 120/80. Mercury is simply a visible liquid used to show the difference between liquid and pressure. When pressure is increased, the mercury is pushed up the scale of the blood pressure machine (the *sphygmomanometer* – see **Measurement of blood pressure** in Chapter 2) and readings can be taken in millimetres or mm for short. The mercury sphygmomanometer used by doctors is similar to the mercury barometer.

I know that the heart beats automatically, but what, if anything, keeps it going?

The heart gets its instructions rather like an electric circuit (Figure 1.3). There is a master switch called the *sinus node* which speeds up and slows down depending on your body's needs. If you are feeling emotional, or running, it goes faster; if you are resting or sleeping, it goes slower.

The sinus node sends messages to a junction box (the *atrioventricular node* or AV node) which regulates the electric impulses before allowing them through into the wires that supply the left heart muscle (ventricle) known as the *left bundle*, or the right ventricle known as the *right bundle*. In this way, if some problem develops so that the control switch races away, the junction box protects your heart by not allowing it to go out of

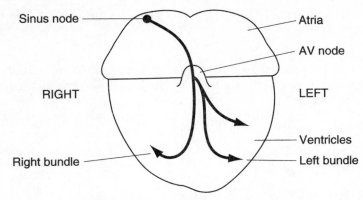

Figure 1.3 The 'electrics' of the heart.

control. Normal impulses start in the sinus node, travel via the atrioventricular node to the 'bundles of wires' that supply the left or right ventricle. The right bundle is single, whilst the left bundle divides into branches (Figure 1.3).

What can go wrong with my heart?

Various things can go wrong with your heart:

- a problem with the pump – the muscle might become weak (thin) or too thick (*hypertrophy*);

- damage to your valves – they might become narrow or develop leaks;

- your coronary arteries might become narrowed or blocked; or

- the 'electrics' might fail – they might short circuit and go too fast or too slow or alternate between fast and slow.

More than one thing can happen at once and one problem can lead to another. This book will explain that there is plenty that you can do to prevent or deal with the problems that occur.

The heart may also be faulty from birth. This condition is known as *congenital* (present at birth, by chance) *heart disease* and can occasionally be inherited (passed on from your parents through your genes).

I am 46 and sometimes feel odd sensations in my chest. Are these to do with my heart? How will I know if I have a heart problem?

The main symptoms people get are:

- chest pain
- breathlessness
- palpitations
- blackouts (less commonly).

If your heart muscle weakens, then you may feel tired or 'washed out', feeling as though you have 'heavy legs' or thinking 'everything is an effort'. Of course, there may be other causes for these symptoms and your doctor will be able to sort them out.

What is the commonest heart problem for me to watch out for?

Coronary artery disease (hardening or narrowing of the arteries to the heart) is the most common problem. The next chapters deal with each condition in turn, describing what the problem is and what treatment is available.

What is the pericardium?

The heart is covered by a thin silky smooth lining called the *pericardium* (peri-car-dee-um). It is known as the *pericardial sac*. Sometimes it becomes inflamed and, instead of being silky, it becomes more like sandpaper and, if the heart rubs against it, it will be painful. Fluid can accumulate in the sac compressing the heart (*pericardial effusion*) leading to breathlessness and a low blood pressure. The fluid can be removed under a local anaesthetic to give instant relief. Inflammation of the pericardium is known as *pericarditis*.

2
Coronary artery disease

Coronary artery disease is caused by a hardening or narrowing of your arteries to the heart The medical term is *atheroma* or *atherosclerosis*. Patches of the inner lining of the arteries become furred up from a mixture of fat, cholesterol and cells deposited in the wall. Veins do not 'fur up' unless asked to do the work of arteries, for example after a bypass operation (see ***Bypass surgery*** in Chapter 3). If you think of the artery as a three-lane motorway, the narrowed part of the artery is like a lane of the motorway being coned off; the traffic is slowed down as it tries to filter into the lanes that are open – a bit like the restricted flow of blood. The patches of narrowing are called *plaque* (pronounced *plack*), so you may hear doctors refer to *atheromatous plaque* or plaque disease. Plaque may cause a progressive narrowing of your arteries, restricting blood flow and causing angina (see Chapter 3), or it may rupture or tear causing clots to form, which totally block the artery, and this can lead to a heart attack. The major causes of atheroma developing are:

- raised cholesterol level;
- cigarette smoking, and
- high blood pressure.

Usually symptoms develop leading to a diagnosis of angina, heart attack or heart failure. Sadly, occasionally, the first evidence may be when someone dies suddenly from a heart attack, but thankfully there is usually a warning and it is important to understand what the warning signs are.

There are some factors in a person's life called *risk factors*. People with risk factors have an increased chance of developing a particular condition. For example, working with asbestos or down a coal mine increases the chance (or *risk*) of developing lung disease and is thus considered a risk factor. Risk factors for coronary artery disease can be divided into those that can be avoided and those that cannot (Table 2.1). Risk factors for coronary disease are like penalty points on a driving licence, only they multiply rather than add up – smoking may give you 3 penalty points and high blood pressure 3 penalty points, but both

Table 2.1 Avoidable and unavoidable risk factors for heart disease

Avoidable	Unavoidable
Cigarette smoking	Male sex
High blood pressure	Family history
High cholesterol	Diabetes (to some extent)
Obesity	Age (getting older)
Lack of exercise	
Stress	

risk factors at the same time may give you 9 penalty points; if you also have 3 penalty points for a high cholesterol level, then your penalty points may multiply to 27 in total.

Are there any risk factors that I can't change?

Your parents, your race (people from the Indian subcontinent have more coronary disease, African Caribbeans less) your age and your sex may increase your risks. Having a family history of heart disease, being a male and getting older means that you need to take more care. But remember that you can lessen many of your risk factors and improve your chances of not developing heart problems.

Prevention is always the best medicine so the first part of this chapter looks at what puts you at risk of developing coronary artery disease, and then how it can be prevented or treated.

Risks of smoking

I have smoked since my teens just as my father and grand-father did. My father is still alive and my grandfather lived until he was 65. What are my risks of heart disease?

There is overwhelming evidence that smoking causes hardening of the coronary arteries as well as hardening of your arteries to the brain and legs; this hardening leads to narrowed arteries and thus poor blood flow to your heart. It also leads to chronic lung diseases as well as lung cancer, and increases your chances of developing a stomach ulcer. Whilst some people escape the consequences of cigarette smoking, the majority do not.

There is a lot of talk about the harmful effects of passive smoking. Can other people's smoke really harm me?

Smoking harms any non-smokers who are breathing in the same air as a smoker, increasing their chance of heart and lung disease.

It may also cause sore red eyes, headaches and make asthma worse. This has become known as *passive smoking*. Children brought up in a household of smokers suffer more infections and disease, compared to those who live in non-smoking households.

The government gives us dire warnings about smoking but I know many people who smoke who are in their seventies or eighties. Are the statistics regarding the harmful effects of smoking really as bad as the press makes out?

Yes. Smoking causes one in five deaths in our population and at least a third of these are due to heart disease. This means that, in the UK, smoking kills 100 000 people a year. It kills 90% of the 40 000 who die from lung cancer, 75% of the 20 000 who die from chronic lung disease such as emphysema, and 25% of the 170 000 who die each year from coronary artery disease. Smoking respects no one – it is an equal opportunity killer attacking both sexes and all races. Out of the total number of people who smoke, a quarter will die early as a result, losing an average 10–15 years of life. Worldwide, smoking kills three million people a year. This is predicted to increase to 10 million by 2025, which means that 200 million of today's children and teenagers will be killed by tobacco. Add these to today's adults and we get a staggering half a billion of the world's population being killed by tobacco – 250 million dying young (aged 35–69 years) and each person losing 20 years of expected life. Many people die only after a long disabling disease.

I have changed to a low-tar brand of cigarettes, with a filter. Why will smoking be so harmful to me now?

Components of tobacco, such as tars, are harmful to your health but the main cause is the nicotine in cigarettes as this is an addictive drug. Nicotine increases your heart rate and blood pressure making your heart work harder, whilst at the same time narrowing the arteries. Oxygen is removed from the blood and replaced with carbon monoxide. Carbon monoxide reduces the ability of the blood to carry oxygen and, in heavy smokers, may reduce it by as much as 50%. We have all read of tragedies caused by faulty gas heaters – carbon monoxide build-up is the cause. This means that there is less energy circulating to your heart to cope with the demands that nicotine places on it. The carbon monoxide level in the blood after smoking one cigarette exceeds the legal limit for pollution allowed in industry by eight times. Low tar cigarettes are nice in theory, because it is the tar in cigarettes that causes lung cancer, but actually they make matters worse in that most low tar smokers inhale deeper and increase their carbon monoxide and nicotine blood levels.

Smoking can cause roughening of the smooth lining of your arteries (the *endothelium*) and this may lead to the development of narrowed areas in the arteries caused by fat being deposited there. Smoking lowers the good cholesterol known as the high density lipoprotein (HDL) (see the section on **Risks of high cholesterol levels**) and increases the blood ingredient (*fibrinogen*) that promotes clotting. Smoking therefore not only causes hardening of your arteries but increases the chance of clots forming on the narrowed areas and thus a heart attack.

I have tried again and again to give up smoking. Are there any 'safe' cigarettes?

No. All cigarettes, 'light' or not, are just as harmful to your heart. Filters have no advantages and may actually increase the carbon monoxide inhaled. Changing to low tar/nicotine cigarettes may reduce your risk of lung cancer, but not heart disease, and it is heart disease that is the major killer.

I cannot stop smoking. Would it help if I just cut down on my smoking?

Yes, but there is no such thing as safe smoking. Smoking five cigarettes a day doubles your risk of heart disease and smoking 20 a day increases your risk by at least 10 times. Reducing the number of cigarettes smoked helps, but quitting is better.

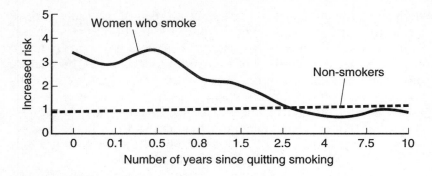

Figure 2.1 Women who smoke have almost four times as great a risk of heart attack but, three years after quitting, the risk is the same as for non-smokers. Solid line = women who smoke; dotted line = non-smokers.

Both my husband and I smoke one pack of cigarettes a day. I have recently read that women are as much at risk as men. Is this true?

Yes and, if anything, more so (Figure 2.1). Women seem to be more sensitive to the effects of cigarettes, so for a similar number smoked (20 per day) you are twice as likely as your husband to develop coronary artery disease. Smoking is especially dangerous if you are on the contraceptive pill, particularly if you are aged over 35 years or have been continuously on the pill for 5 years or more (see section on *Women and coronary artery disease*).

If I could stop smoking, would this do any real good?

Four to five years after quitting smoking, your risk of heart disease will be the same as for a non-smoker. Stopping smoking is one of the most important actions you can make – not starting is the best educational message of all (Figure 2.2). The benefit to your lungs takes longer – about 20 years.

I am 58 and have been smoking for many years. Is it ever too late to stop?

No. The benefit to your heart is rapid and helps you, no matter what your age.

My girlfriend has suggested that I change to a pipe as she is convinced that pipes and cigars are safer than cigarettes. Is this true?

Smoke from pipes and cigars contains a higher concentration of tar and nicotine compared with cigarettes, but pipe and cigar smokers usually inhale less than cigarette smokers so the risks are less, but they are still greater than in non-smokers. Cigarette smokers who switch to a pipe usually inhale the smoke automatically, thereby not significantly reducing their risks. Studies have shown that smokers, who switch to pipes and cigars and don't inhale, reduce their risks of lung cancer and heart disease by 50%, but the risk is still 50% higher than quitting altogether. However, by not inhaling, pipe and cigar smokers increase the risk to non-smokers from passive smoking. The best option is not to smoke at all. The principal reason pipe smokers have less risk is that they spend most of their time trying to light the pipe rather than puffing on it!

Figure 2.2 Cigarette smoking is the biggest risk factor for sudden death. The best advice is: If you smoke – QUIT; if you don't smoke – DON'T START.

I have tried to stop smoking but always lapse. What can I do to quit smoking and avoid the temptations?

Stopping smoking *is* difficult but it is the biggest single improvement to your health that you, as a smoker, can make. Some people find that a book on quitting gives them the confidence that they need to actually stop. There are some suggestions on book titles that may be helpful in Appendix 3.

Cutting down is a help but only if your aim is to stop completely (see question above). Remember that after 3–5 years you will have your heart's health back. Here are some guidelines to help you:

- Make a list of your reasons for stopping, keep it with you and read it every day. The best reasons are:
  - it is bad for my health;
  - the cough is unpleasant;
  - my clothes always smell;
  - it is expensive;
  - I cannot taste my food;
  - non-smokers are upset by my smoking.
- Set a day to stop or take part in a sponsored 'stop' with friends or business colleagues.
- Take time for exercise, drink plenty of water and have plenty of fresh fruit to hand (not cakes or biscuits).
- Each day place the money saved to one side and put it into a savings account. After 1 week you will have saved around £30, by 1 month £120, and by 6 months £720, which you can spend on a well-earned holiday. Put another way, if you place the price of a packet of cigarettes at around £4 per day into an individual savings account (ISA), after 20 years the fund could be worth £44 100 (at 6% interest). In a pension plan, it could give you £4,350 (at 7% interest) per year in extra annual income! Of course, if you carry on smoking, you may never reach your pensionable age.

- Be disciplined and don't talk yourself into smoking 'to calm me down'. If the craving is unbearable, go for a brisk walk, relax with a hot bath and drink plenty of water.

- Think positively.

- Don't carry matches or a lighter.

- Go to the dentist and have your teeth cleaned to get rid of the tobacco stains.

- Keep being positive, keep reading your reasons for quitting, reward yourself with a treat after your first week of not smoking – you've saved enough money, so go ahead!

- Avoid certain activities that are linked with smoking:

  – Try to avoid alcohol and take a drink that is not associated with smoking, such as a tomato juice.

  – After a meal, instead of a cigarette, clean the table, wash up, brush your teeth and go for a walk.

  – Do not have cigarettes in the car; have chewing gum to hand instead.

- Avoid smoky restaurants or public houses.

- Visit places where smoking is not allowed (library, museum, art gallery, cinema).

- Tell your smoking friends that you will be unavailable other than on the 'phone, unless they are giving up as well.

- Keep your hands busy (fiddle with paper clips, write a letter, do the crossword, clean the car, help in the garden or with the housework).

- Use sugarless chewing gum to replace the urge to put a cigarette in your mouth.

- Take deep breaths, relax your muscles, and think of anything but cigarettes, for example your holiday plans or a previous happy experience.

- Remove everything from the house that reminds you of cigarettes: get rid of your ashtrays and matches, then have a spring clean to remove all the smell and stains of smoking, open the windows and let the fresh air circulate.

If you tell yourself you don't want to smoke rather than wishing you could smoke, you can reinforce this by noticing that your breath is better, your clothes are cleaner, the car smells better, food tastes again and that early morning cough has improved or stopped! Remember the 10 million people who have already broken the habit. The first few days are always the worst, so it does get easier!

I've given up smoking but I am afraid that I might begin again. Will it put me back to square one if I start again?

Try to avoid the urge but, if you do slip, don't despair: you can get back the ground you've lost, but you must act quickly. It is not a crime, you are not a failure, and you must not feel guilty. Look for the reason (Were you tense or stressed? Were you upset or angry? Were you in a situation that you automatically associated with smoking?) and then take action to avoid it happening again.

I have heard that meditation can help people to stop smoking. Do you think it works and is it worth the effort?

A lot of people benefit from learning to relax and meditate. It is particularly useful in times of stress. Relaxation tapes are available and can be helpful, as can relaxing music.

A friend of mine went to an acupuncturist to help her stop smoking and she has not smoked now for some months. I have also read that hypnosis can help. Do you think that any of these methods is any good?

There is no trial (research) evidence that acupuncture or hypnosis is effective in helping people stop smoking. However, if you are struggling, it may be worth trying either or both as they are popular with smokers and people can be helped by unproven methods. Make sure that you go to registered practitioners and keep and open mind. Always enquire about the cost before treatment begins.

I don't do much exercise. Would exercise help me to give up smoking?

Exercise is very helpful. It not only improves your overall physical condition, but it is also a great way of relieving stress and improving your mood. It takes your mind off cigarettes as well as helping to control your appetite and weight. Before you exercise, practise deep breathing and repeat this as you cool down afterwards. Dynamic exercise is best and this includes walking as briskly as possible, cycling, swimming and playing tennis or golf (see Chapter 10).

I know people who have given up smoking, but then put on weight. How can I avoid this?

People who smoke are on average 3–4 kg (7–8 lb) lighter than non-smokers. It is, however, the wrong way to stay slim. When you stop it doesn't automatically mean your weight will go up, but gaining 1 kg (2–3 lb) is not as important as quitting cigarettes.

Weight is gained when you eat more than you burn up. The trick is to watch what you eat and take up regular exercise. You need to plan positively not to let it happen.

Eat fresh fruit and vegetables, avoid cakes chocolate and biscuits, use whole-grain cereals, porridge without sugar, pasta and bread, and drink plenty of water or low calorie drinks. You will not control your weight unless you match your intake with regular exercise – you must do both (see Chapters 9 and 10). Think of it as a lifestyle change, not a 'diet'.

It is not a good idea to stop smoking just as you go on holiday, as there will be a temptation to overeat anyway. Weigh yourself no more than once a week, at the same time of day and in the same or no clothing, to monitor your progress. Try not to become obsessed by weight. Do not start to smoke if your weight goes up; watch what you are eating and take plenty of exercise.

I've not yet tried quitting as I am frankly unable to cope with going 'cold turkey'. What can I expect as withdrawal symptoms when I stop smoking?

There is often a worsening of the smoker's cough until all the rubbish is out of your lungs. You may feel thirsty, in which case drink water and avoid caffeinated drinks and excess alcohol. Some people become constipated and hungry, and this is helped by fresh fruit and a high fibre diet (see Chapter 9). Some people become anxious, irritable and have difficulty concentrating – these feelings may last up to 4 weeks but are worse in the first 2 weeks. Drink plenty of water and take regular exercise; try to fill your time with positive activities (see the question above).

I have seen adverts for nicotine gum and patches. I smoke about 20 a day. Would nicotine replacement help me?

Some people are so addicted to nicotine that they need to be weaned off – they tend to be the people who need their first cigarette within 30 minutes of waking in the morning.

There are five sorts of nicotine replacements:

- The **patch** is like a thin elastoplast, which slowly gives out nicotine through the skin. It does not help if you have a sudden craving but, if you normally smoke steadily over a day, it will almost certainly suit your needs. Studies have shown that people using the patch, compared to those using a dummy patch (with no nicotine), had twice the success rate in stopping smoking. Patches come in different strengths, and heavy smokers (over 20 a day) may need to start high, weaning down to lower strengths over 2–4 weeks. Common products are Boots and Nicorette (5, 10 and 15 mg) and Nicotinell and NiQuitin CQ (7, 14 and 21 mg).

- Nicotine gum, inhalator, tablet or nasal spray help you respond to a sudden craving because they act quickly – so you may be more likely to need these if you smoke in response to sudden stress. Boots, Nicorette and Nicotinell **gum** (flavoured or plain) come in two strengths, 2 and 4 mg, and can be bought in chemist shops. Again, heavy smokers may need to start with the 4mg strength; 8–12 pieces of either strength each day are recommended starting doses.

- The Nicorette **nasal spray** is prescription only (one spray each nostril up to twice an hour for 16 hours in every 24).

- Boots and Nicorette **inhalators** consist of a mouthpiece and replaceable nicotine cartridge – you should suck the nicotine vapour into the mouth (it does not reach the lungs). Each cartridge provides up to three 20-minute periods of intense use, and you may need 6–12 cartridges a day for 8 weeks, reducing to zero over the next 4 weeks. These can be bought in chemist shops.

- The Nicorette **tablet** (Microtab) is placed under the tongue and dissolves over 30 minutes, providing 1mg of nicotine from a 2mg tablet. You may need one or two hourly at first, and they can be bought in chemist shops.

The instructions must be followed carefully, and any concerns should be discussed with your family doctor or chemist. Do not use nicotine products if you are pregnant or breastfeeding.

Are there any side effects to the nicotine preparations?

For most people, side effects are not a problem. The gum may be awkward if you have dentures, and the patches may cause the skin to itch, so you may need to move them to a different place each day. The nasal spray may irritate the nose and throat and make your eyes water; the inhalator may cause a cough or irritation of the throat. The tablet can mildly irritate the mouth, but this tends to wear off with use. Sleep disturbance, vivid dreams, flushing or rashes, and nausea sometimes occur. Nicotine can upset a stomach (peptic) ulcer, so, if you are on treatment for an ulcer, check with your doctor first. If you have a history of heart attack, stroke, high blood pressure, diabetes or hardening of the arteries generally, check with your doctor first. If you are taking warfarin, inform your clinic, as there may be an interaction between the two drugs. Too much nicotine may make you feel sick, so do not smoke at the same time as using gum or patches. Whilst combining nicotine preparations is not recommended by the manufacturers, some studies have shown improved success rates when the gum and patches, or the nasal spray and patches, are combined. Only do this after getting your doctor's advice.

Can I become addicted to the nicotine patches?

This is not a problem with the patches. However, the gum, spray, tablet or inhalator, which deal with cravings, may need to be used for over a year. When you are trying to stop using nicotine replacements, wean off gently to avoid a withdrawal reaction. You will be more successful if you combine nicotine replacement with the support of smokers' clinics and family, rather than going it alone.

How much do these products cost?

Approximate costs for 3 months paying yourself are:

- Boots 2 mg gum £120

- Nicorette inhalator £300

- Nicorette spray £110

- Nicorette patches up to £150.

You will save your money and your life for many years ahead – think of this cost as a down payment towards better health. The good news is that nicotine replacement therapy is now approved by the National Health Service and is regarded as the drug treatment of choice. The family doctor and the patient must follow an agreed protocol and set a target stop date before a prescription is allowed.

I have been trying to find a support group – can they help me?

They certainly help. You will feel less alone, get support and help from others and be amongst people all trying to succeed. Phone QUIT on 020 7388 5775, or check with your local health authority for locations. QUITLINE (0800 00 22 00) provides trained counsellors to give advice, support and encouragement (see Appendix 2).

There are now NHS helplines in England and Wales (0800 169 0169), Scotland (0800 84 84 84) and Northern Ireland (028 9066 3281). Also try www.sickofsmoking.com to see what other smokers say.

Are herbal cigarettes or dummy cigarettes worth trying?

Dummy cigarettes, such as Crave Away, Flowers or Everlasting Cigarettes, are neither harmful nor proven to be effective. Herbal cigarettes do not contain nicotine but still expose your body to tar and carbon monoxide, and are of no proven value.

Would it be better if I used a filter?

Filters can be a good idea, but unfortunately do not work for most people. Nicobrevin may help in the first weeks but should not be relied on as a long-term prop. It should be avoided if you are pregnant. Note that filters remove some of the tar but little of the risk of heart disease!

Why do some people smoke like chimneys but live a long life all the same?

Most people know someone like this. It is all about statistics: if 90% of people die from smoking, then 10% won't. The point is that the odds are against you, and trying to get away with it, or believing it can't happen to you, is courting disaster.

If someone introduced a product onto the market now that was addictive, removed oxygen from your blood, caused blood clotting, heart attacks and lung cancer, do you think they would get a licence?

I have heard a lot about Zyban. Does it help stop smoking and how does it work?

Zyban is the trade name for the drug buproprion. It is a drug used to treat depression but it was also found to help people stop smoking. How it does this is unclear but it seems to reduce the urge for nicotine and is effective for some people. It should be started 1–2 weeks before the target stop date and continued for 7–9 weeks after. It should not be used in anyone with a history of seizures (fits) or eating disorders. It also has the potential to react with some drugs. Zyban should only be used after careful discussion with your family doctor – it is available on NHS prescription.

I had a heart attack a year ago when I was 61. Is it too late to stop smoking?

It is never too late. Stopping smoking after a heart attack reduces by half your chance of having another one in the next 5 years. Stopping smoking after a heart bypass operation reduces your chances of a bypass failure over the next 10–15 years and helps prevent further disease developing.

What is a smoking cessation clinic – is it worth a try?

Special clinics and specially trained nurses and smoking cessation advisors provide support and achieve high success rates in smoking cessation. Support is usually given in groups over 6 weeks and most services also offer one-to-one counselling. Clinics take direct referrals from those wanting to stop (in a walk-in service) as well as working in partnership with family doctors. They are recommended for heavily dependent smokers needing intensive support or pregnant women especially. However, they are available to all either in a clinic setting or as part of a local primary care service. As stopping smoking is so important – if you are having any difficulty, certainly give them a try.

Risks of high blood pressure

Facts and figures

Can you tell me more about blood pressure? Why is it serious if it becomes high?

We need a blood pressure to send blood around our bodies (see Chapter 1). It is needed to overcome the resistance of the smaller blood vessels. The arteries in the body have muscle in their walls to give them tone. If this muscle is supple, the arteries can relax, their size or width increases and blood flows more easily. Think of the artery like a garden hose pipe: if you turn the tap on, water flows easily – now clamp the pipe to reduce its size by half and water will need more pressure to get through to give the same flow. In a similar way, the heart pumps the blood through the arteries but, if your arteries get smaller, the pressure will need to rise in order to force the blood through (Figure 2.3). The top pressure known as the *systolic pressure* (pronounced *sis-tol-ick*) is the pressure created by your heart beating and coincides with your pulse, and the bottom pressure known as the *diastolic pressure* (pronounced *die-a-stol-ick*) is the reading when your heart is relaxing. The readings should not be more than 140/90 mmHg (Hg is the symbol for mercury which is in the column of the blood pressure machine).

Blood pressure can clearly be raised (e. g. 220/120) (when it known as *hypertension* – see below) or normal (e. g. 120/80), but there are areas where it is borderline, and you need regular checks to keep an eye on it. A pressure consistently above 160/90 mmHg should be investigated but age should be taken into account as well. At 80 years this figure might be okay, but at 30 years it would not be. So although doctors talk generally of blood

Systolic (peak pressure)

Healthy systolic pressure
is no more than 140

Healthy diastolic pressure
is no more than 90

Diastolic (trough)

Systolic pressure
over 140 indicates
hypertension

Diastolic pressure
over 90 indicates
hypertension

(a) Normal pressure

(b) Higher pressure needed

Figure 2.3 (a) Healthy arteries are elastic and blood flows easily without meeting a resistance. (b) Arteries can lose their elasticity for unknown reasons or suffer from disease or hardening with age. They then become less able to relax and a higher pressure is needed to force the blood through.

pressure, any decision to investigate or treat will be made on a very individual basis.

Hypertension (pronounced *hi-per-ten-shun*) is the medical word for a high blood pressure. *Hyper* means too much, and *tension* refers to the pressure. You may be asked to attend a hypertension clinic or a screening clinic to keep a check on your blood pressure.

What causes high blood pressure?

In the vast majority of cases there is no single cause, just as there is no single cause for people being short or tall. The medical name is *essential* or *primary hypertension*. Tests may be done to check the kidneys, adrenal gland and heart. Some people's blood pressure is raised as a side effect of their medication, particularly anti-arthritis medications. Always tell your doctor or practice nurse what medicines your have (including complementary or herbal medicines) or, preferably, bring along any that you are taking to show your doctor.

You may have been told that you have *secondary hypertension* – this is the term used when a cause for your high blood pressure has been found (this happens in only 5% of cases). The normal or target pressure is 140/90 mmHg or less and in people with diabetes 130/80 mmHg.

What tests can I expect to have if my blood pressure is found to be raised?

The heart may be checked with an ECG (see under *Tests* in Chapter 3) or echocardiogram (see under *Tests* in Chapter 5). A chest X-ray may be taken to look at the heart and lungs. Blood and water (urine) tests will look for any signs of anaemia (low blood count) or kidney problems, and your urine may be collected for 24 hours to see if there is too much adrenaline coming from your adrenal gland. Sometimes a scan or X-ray is taken of the kidneys.

I am not too sure what the adrenal glands are for? Can you explain their purpose?

The adrenal glands sit on top of your kidneys. They produce adrenaline. This is a hormone which speeds up your heart when you exert yourself or are emotionally excited or very frightened (white with fear), and you feel your heart pounding. Adrenaline keeps your blood pressure up if you are shocked or losing blood. Too much adrenaline that is not needed, for example in a person who is not exercising, will keep the blood pressure high unnecessarily. A tumour of the adrenal gland can do this and, although they are very rare, we check the blood or urine for excess adrenaline in younger people. If an excess is found and a tumour shown on a scan, it can be removed surgically.

My wife and I went to the doctors to get our blood pressures checked. Hers was different to mine. Why?

Blood pressure can change from person to person and also in the same person. Blood pressure constantly changes within a normal range depending on what you are doing.

During physical work your muscles need a greater supply of food and, to meet this extra demand, your blood flow has to be increased. To achieve this, your heart must beat faster and your blood pressure rises.

Blood pressure is lowest at night when you are asleep, but even then there are fluctuations which are presumably due to the influence of dreams. During the day the fluctuations are greater and more frequent and reflect the sort of work you are doing. Mental as well as physical stress can increase your blood pressure.

From this you will see that a doctor may need to take several readings of your blood pressure to make sure that a diagnosis of high blood pressure is a true reflection, and not due to an isolated event that could be responsible for a temporary rise in pressure. For this reason your doctor may ask you to call back to the surgery over a period of a few days or weeks in order to eliminate any temporary cause for the high level.

You can help your doctor in this respect by arriving early for your appointment, so as to avoid a rush, or worrying that you will be late. When you arrive in the surgery, relax as much as possible, because it is important to your doctor, when he is judging the level of blood pressure, to know that you are rested and calm at the time the measurement is taken (see next question).

When I went to the clinic to have my blood pressure checked, I was told that I probably had 'white coat hypertension'. What is this?

This is a high reading caused by anxiety or stress when you visit your doctor (who may be wearing a white coat!). At other times your blood pressure is usually normal. It may be worth checking the readings at home and during the day with a blood pressure machine that can be worn while you are walking about (an *ambulatory* machine). (See the question later on about this.) Do several readings with your own or a borrowed machine. Blood pressure often rises under stress; throughout the day we are exposed to many stresses, so if several elevated readings occur because of environmental stress, treatment will be of value. If no elevated readings occur, your doctor should monitor your pressure regularly anyway, because we don't know if white coat hypertension is a warning for true hypertension in the future. You cannot afford to be complacent.

When I was 16, my blood pressure was lower than it is now that I am 45. Is this OK?

Yes, as a natural part of growing old, your arteries tend to lose their elastic properties to some degree. Also, the walls of your arteries tend to thicken after middle age and, consequently, the internal diameter of the vessel is slightly reduced (the hose pipe gets narrower). All these changes require a very slight increase in blood pressure, which is perfectly normal as you get older.

What are the dangers if I can't get my high blood pressure down?

If a raised blood pressure is left untreated over a 12-year period, you are more likely to die from this risk than if you had been treated. Other statistics about raised blood pressure are:

- It is present in 70% of people who have a stroke.

- It increases the risk of coronary heart disease by 2–3 times for men and women.

- It causes heart and kidney failure.

- It causes hardening of the arteries to the legs resulting in pain on walking owing to poor blood flow (the medical term for this is *claudication*, pronounced *claw-di-ca-shun*).

- It is responsible for a third of all heart diseases.

- It causes seven out of 10 strokes in women and four out of 10 in men.

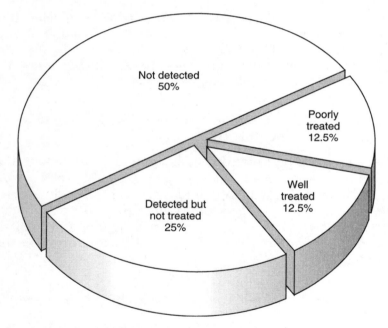

Figure 2.4 The rule of halves in people with high blood pressure: they remain poorly detected and poorly treated. Half the people with a high blood pressure do not know that they have it (not detected); half who have it may not have been told or may not have attended for treatment; half of those on treatment are not well controlled and finally half of those on treatment are properly treated and have normal pressures as a result – not a good record!

- In the UK, 300 people die as a result of a high blood pressure every 6 weeks and most of these deaths are avoidable – if a jumbo jet with 300 people on board crashed every 6 weeks, something would be done about it!

Are there any specific risk factors for high blood pressure that might apply to me?

A high blood pressure is more common:

- when someone in your family has had high blood pressure;
- if you are an African Caribbean;
- if you are aged over 60 years of age;
- if you are very overweight;
- if you drink heavily;
- if you eat a lot of salt;
- if you had a high blood pressure in pregnancy, or pre-eclampsia;
- if you have a lot of stress in your life.

I have read about the rule of halves, but did not understand it. Could you explain?

This is a medical paradox but in reality it demonstrates some alarming facts about blood pressure and lack of treatment.

- Half the people with high BP have not been diagnosed.
- Half of those diagnosed have not been treated.
- Half of those treated have not got their blood pressure under control.
- Half of those treated are well treated; and so
- Only one-eighth of people with high blood pressure are being properly treated (Figure 2.4).

So the responsibility is yours to keep nagging your doctor or practice nurse to check your blood pressure, whenever you go to the surgery. You must take charge of your own health.

How would I know if my blood pressure was raised?

Most people feel nothing until there is a problem, which is why it is known as the silent enemy. It is thought that half the people with high blood pressure do not know they have it, because they cannot feel it and a doctor has not checked it. It is therefore important to have a blood pressure check every few years if it is normal, or more frequently if it is slightly raised or 'borderline'. If you go to your doctor for another reason, ask for it to be checked then.

Measurement of blood pressure

I have often seen home blood pressure monitoring machines in high street chemists, but they are pricey. Are they any good?

Some are, but others are not accurate or reliable. Ask your doctor for advice on which one to buy and then get it checked against the doctor's machine. Ask the nurse if you are not sure how to use it – go through a practice run in the surgery. Some doctors can loan you a machine for a couple of days. This is the best option because the most reliable electronic machines are the most expensive – a medical centre can buy one or two and keep an eye on their accuracy by regular checks, making sure the cuff is the right size and the batteries fresh. Digital monitors have a cuff, which inflates and deflates at the touch of a button. The Omron has been approved and validated but, for up-to-date advice, contact the British Hypertension Society (Appendix 2).

How is blood pressure measured in the clinic?

Your doctor or nurse takes the blood pressure with an instrument called a *sphygmomanometer* (often abbreviated to *sphyg*) (Figure 2.5). It is pronounced *s-fig-mo-man-omeater*. The Greek word for pulse is *sphygmos* and it is the appearance and disappearance of the pulse at the elbow that the doctor or nurse listens for.

While your arm is relaxed and resting on a desk or supported by the doctor or nurse, a rubber cuff is wound round your upper arm just above the elbow. If your arm is large, a big cuff will be used. The cuff is attached to a column of mercury. The cuff is inflated by air being pumped into the cuff; you will feel a squeezing feeling. The pressure in the cuff is increased until the blood flow to your hand is cut off (you may feel a tingling or numbness). Whilst the doctor listens with a stethoscope to the

Figure 2.5 Getting your blood pressure checked in the surgery.

artery at the elbow (the *brachial artery*, pronounced *brake-e-al*), the pressure in the cuff is lowered. The level of mercury shown in the column when the blood begins to flow again (felt as a thumping) is measured as the *systolic pressure* and, when no noises are heard (you don't feel this), it is measured as the diastolic pressure. Always ask what your reading is and keep your own records.

How often should my blood pressure be checked?

Once a year if it is normal – try and make a note in your diary to make an appointment for the following year. If it is raised, your doctor will take several readings and keep an eye on it until it is normal. Your blood pressure will then be checked at regular intervals, usually every 3–6 months. Make sure that you ask for this measurement at least twice a year.

My doctor tells me that my systolic pressure is very high, although the diastolic pressure is normal. Does this matter?

It used to be thought that only the diastolic blood pressure rise was important, but modern research has shown that in people over the age of 45 years, the rise in systolic blood pressure over the normal of 140, and certainly over 160, is an important cause of subsequent heart disease and strokes. Treatment of this rise in systolic blood pressure is an important factor in reducing the risk of these serious complications.

Self-help

My mother had high blood pressure and she suffered a stroke when she was 65. Can I avoid having hypertension myself?

First of all, if someone in your family has had high blood pressure, make sure that you and your relatives have regular

check-ups. Although you may feel no benefit now, you may help
to prevent illness in the future, so adopt a positive approach – for
yourself and those you care about. Other ways of helping yourself
include:

- a healthy diet (see Chapter 9)
- exercise (see Chapter 10)
- avoiding getting overweight
- avoiding excess alcohol
- avoiding eating excess salt.

**I'm 62 and my doctor is making me cut down on salt as she
says that I am getting more sensitive to salt. What does
this mean?**

People over 60 years, African Caribbeans and American Blacks
have been found to have less tolerance to too much salt. Salt-
sensitive people can lower their blood pressure by 5–10mmHg by
cutting down on salt. Most, however, get a benefit of up to
4mmHg, but every little bit helps to lower blood pressure and
reduce the need for medication.

**My husband has been told that he has a high blood
pressure. The doctor gave him a diet sheet. How can a
better diet help him?**

Your husband should not overeat as, apart from anything else,
this will make him put on weight, and being overweight is a major
risk factor for and cause of high blood pressure. The single most
important thing anybody with high blood pressure can do to help
themselves is to lose weight. In some lucky people the raised
pressure disappears completely and, in others, fewer tablets may
be needed. If your husband is overweight, a reducing diet to get
him to an optimum weight is an essential part of treatment.
Losing 1 kg in weight could take two points off his blood pressure
reading, so losing 3 kg (half a stone) can make a borderline

Table 2.2 Common drugs for raised blood pressure

Generic (real) name	Trade name (can vary in different countries)
Diuretics	
bendrofluazide	Aprinox
chlorthalidone	Hygroton
hydrochlorothiazide	Hydrenox, Hydrosaluric
indapamide	Natrilix
Potassium-sparing diuretics	
amiloride	Usually in combination
triamterine	Dytac
spironolactone	Aldactone
Beta-blockers	
acebutolol	Sectral
atenolol	Tenormin, Totamol
bisoprolol	Emcor, Monocor
carvedilol	Eucardic
celiprolol	Celectol
labetalol	Trandate
metoprolol	Betaloc, Lopresor
nebivolol	Nebilet
pindolol	Visken
propranolol	Beta-Prograne, Inderal
timolol	Betim, Blocadren
Calcium antagonists	
amlodipine	Istin
diltiazem	Tildiem, Adizem, Dilzem
felodipine	Plendil
isradipine	Prescal
lacidipine	Motens
nicardipine	Cardene SR
nifedipine	Adalat, Adalat LA, Cardilate MR, Coracten XL,
nisoldipine	Syscor MR
verapamil	Securon, Cordilox, Univer
ACE inhibitors	
captopril	Capoten, Acepril
cilazapril	Vascace
enalapril	Innovace

Generic (real) name	Trade name (can vary in different countries)
ACE inhibitors (continued)	
fosinopril	Staril
lisinopril	Carace, Zestril
moexipril	Perdix
perindopril	Coversyl
quinapril	Accupro
ramipril	Tritace
trandolapril	Gopten, Odrik
Alpha-blockers	
doxazosin	Cardura
indoramin	Baratol
prazosin	Hypovase
terazosin	Hytrin
Angiotensin II antagonists	
candesartan	Amias
irbesartan	Aprovel
losartan	Cozaar
telmisartan	Micardis
valsartan	Diovan
Combination products	
atenolol + chlorthalidone	Tenoret 50, Tenoretic
atenolol + nifedipine	Tenif, Beta-Adalat
captopril + hydrochlorothiazide	Capozide, Acezide
enalapril + hydrochlorothiazide	Innozide
lisinopril + hydrochlorothiazide	Zestoretic
losartan + hydrochlorothiazide	Cozaar-Comp
metoprolol + hydrochlorothiazide	Co-Betaloc
propranolol + bendrofluazide	Inderetic
perindopril + indapamide	Coversyl Plus
irbesartan + hydrochlorothiazide	Co Aprovel

pressure normal. However, his pressure will still need watching and will go back up again if the weight is put back on. See Chapter 9 for advice on a healthy diet and how to lose weight.

Treatment

I am bitterly disappointed because I have lost weight and reduced my salt intake, but I have been told that my blood pressure is still raised. What should I do?

You will need medication. Lowering your blood pressure to normal removes your chances of having a stroke and protects your heart, brain and kidneys from damage.

The good news is that treatment is very effective. Controlling high blood pressure helps prevent all the problems developing and restores you to a normal life expectancy. We now have many effective medications available to treat hypertension that need to be taken only once a day; if one causes a side effect, there is no need to despair because we have lots of choices and we can always find another drug that lowers the pressure to suit you.

There seem to be a lot of different medications on the market for raised blood pressure. Why have I been given one and not another?

There are various types of medications in common use. Table 2.2 gives a list of the most commonly prescribed medications for raised blood pressure and Table 2.3 lists some of their possible side effects. The drugs have a generic or chemical name and a trade name under which they may be marketed. The trade names vary between countries so always check against the generic name to make sure that you are on the recommended medication.

Diuretics or 'water tablets' are commonly used. They remove excess salt and water from the body. They can also wash out too much potassium (and this may cause cramps) which can be dangerous if digoxin is also being taken. In some people, diuretics cause gout, and if you have diabetes they can raise your blood sugar, upsetting control of your diabetes. Common medications in this group include bendrofluazide (Aprinox), hydrochlorothiazide (Hydrenox, Hydrosaluric) and chlorthalidone (Hygroton) To reduce the loss of potassium, so-called potassium-sparing agents can be prescribed and these include

Table 2.3 Blood pressure-lowering drugs and their possible side effects

Drug type	Possible side effects
Beta-blockers	Cold hands and feet with or without numb feeling (pins and needles); lethargy, poor concentration; heavy legs (like a zombie); wheezing; dry eyes
Diuretics	Impotence; rashes; gout; possible problems for people with diabetes; muscle cramps
Calcium antagonists	Flushing, headaches and dizziness; swollen ankles which may be painful; bloated feeling and constipation
ACE inhibitors	Dry hacking cough; rash; stomach upsets
Alpha-blockers	Tiredness; dizziness; dry mouth
Angiotensin II antagonists	No major or common ones reported
Drugs that act on the brain (e.g. methyldopa, moxonidine)	Weakness, drowsiness, dizziness on standing; dry mouth; depression; impotence

spironolactone (Aldactone), triamterene (Dytac), or amiloride. These two sorts of medications may be combined, e. g. Aldactide, Moduretic or Dyazide, in order to try and get the best results. Diuretics in general are safe and effective and side effects are not common. Fresh fruit is a good way of replacing potassium – a banana a day may do the trick.

Beta-blockers are also frequently prescribed. These act to slow your heart rate and lower your blood pressure by blocking the effects of adrenaline. Commonly used medications are atenolol (Tenormin), metoprolol (Betaloc, Lopresor) and bisoprolol (Monocor). The commonest side effects are cold hands and feet, heavy legs, lethargy and a 'zombie-like' feeling. Beta-blockers may cause wheezing and are not used in people with asthma. They may also hide the signs of a low sugar level in people with Type 1 (insulin-dependent) diabetes. They do not tend to mask the perspiration that goes with a hypoglycaemic attack (low sugar episode), so this warning sign is preserved. If the diabetes is stable and well controlled, they are used, but more often if there is also angina present (see Chapter 3).

As a group, they are useful medications and if you have had a heart attack, you may live longer if you are prescribed them. They can be combined with diuretics for an additive effect and may be available with a diuretic in a single tablet, e. g. Tenoretic.

Calcium antagonists act to expand the arteries, making it easier for blood to flow (widen the hose pipe). They can be used with diuretics and some can be used with beta-blockers (but not verapamil – Securon, Cordilox, Univer – as the heart rate can get dangerously slow). They are helpful if you have asthma, and do not affect the medications that you may be receiving if you have diabetes. Commonly prescribed medications are amlodipine (Istin), diltiazem (Tildiem, Adizem, Dilzem), nifedipine (Adalat), verapamil and felodipine (Plendil). Side effects include water retention (causing swollen ankles and legs), headaches, constipation (especially verapamil), occasional palpitations and sore gums. Impotence is unusual. Again these are useful medications which seem to be of more value in the elderly and African Caribbeans. Older people and African Caribbeans have a different hormone pattern from the kidneys, which makes calcium antagonists more effective.

ACE inhibitors and angiotensin II (AII) antagonists are widely used. ACE stands for angiotensin-converting enzyme. This enzyme is normally present in the body; blocking it causes the blood vessels to relax (the blood pressure falls as it meets less resistance) and reduces salt and water retention. Angiotensin II antagonists act in the same way but at a different point from ACE inhibitors – the end result is the same but the cough side effect of the ACE inhibitors (see below) is avoided.

ACE inhibitors include captopril (Capoten, Acepril), lisinopril (Carace, Zestril) and enalapril (Innovace), whilst the AIIs include losartan (Cozaar) and valsartan (Diovan). They both act much the same way by blocking chemicals that constrict the arteries and retain salt and water. If you have heart failure, ACE inhibitors can lengthen your life and can protect people with diabetes from kidney damage. The main side effect is a dry hacking cough. These are important medications which have few side effects and are not known to interfere with your quality of life, including your sex life. ACE inhibitors have recently been shown to benefit patients with coronary artery disease in the absence of high blood pressure or heart failure.

Alpha-blockers act on nerve receptors to dilate the arteries – this in turn lowers the blood pressure. Prazosin (Hypovase) and doxazosin (Cardura) are the most common ones. They can cause tiredness and dizzy feelings. Their major advantage is the reduction in prostate symptoms in a male. They can be combined with all the other medications and are safe in people with asthma or diabetes.

I read in the newspaper and saw a report on TV that calcium antagonists can be dangerous – is this true?

Unfortunately for reasons that are not clear, there have been scare stories about calcium antagonists. The evidence has been refuted by other researchers who looked at the claims in depth. Very high doses of nifedipine capsules can cause angina because of the speed of action of this preparation, but the capsules are not used routinely and very rarely in high doses. Claims made of an increased risk of heart attack or cancer do not stand up to careful scientific scrutiny –the claims are so devoid of scientific fact that the stories should not have been put out publicly. Much of what has been written about the dangers of calcium antagonists is nonsense and this has upset many patients and doctors. There is no danger if you take long-acting calcium antagonists such as amlodipine, nifedipine LA (long-acting), and diltiazem LA, but you should avoid short-acting formulations such as nifedipine capsules. The calcium antagonist scares are a classical example of media hype with commercial undertones.

Someone told me that one particular medication for blood pressure makes your hair grow – is this true?

Yes. Minoxidil is a very potent treatment used only in severe resistant blood pressure cases. It can make people put on weight because of water retention and is not used routinely for this reason. It also makes your hair grow – this can be an advantage in bald men but is not usually liked by women!

You have not mentioned Aldomet. I am pregnant and my doctor prescribed this medication for my blood pressure. Why did she choose this rather than the others that you have talked about?

Methyldopa (Aldomet) is an old and effective drug for lowering blood pressure but it does have a large number of side effects. It can cause drowsiness, sluggishness, a dry mouth, depression and impotence (see Chapter 8). Because of these effects, it is not used so much these days and has been replaced by more user-friendly medications. However, it is effective and its main use today is for raised blood pressure in pregnancy, as the medication does not cause harm to your baby. It is usually stopped on delivery to reduce the chances of depression following the birth.

I've read about a new medication called Physiotens which was called a breakthrough for blood pressure treatment in my newspaper. Should I get my doctor to put me on it?

Physiotens is the trade names for moxonidine. It acts via the brain and is advised for mild to moderate hypertension if other drugs are not appropriate or are not fully effective. Side effects include dry mouth, headache, fatigue dizziness and sleep disturbance. It has an effective but limited place in treatment.

When I went to see my doctor, he measured my blood pressure and put me on tablets straightaway. Why was this?

If your blood pressure was very high when it was first measured, it would be unlikely that changing your lifestyle alone would help. However, it is worth trying the measures discussed in the section on *Self-help* earlier because these may help to reduce the amount of tablets you need.

I have been feeling tired and lethargic lately. Do you think my tablets are causing the problem?

All medications can cause side effects. We try hard as doctors to prescribe the safest and most convenient medications. If you are concerned that a particular medication is causing a problem, let your doctor know. It may have occurred by chance but it may also be associated with your treatment and a change in your medicine could relieve the symptoms. For instance, if you feel that your sex life has been affected, it may be due to your medications.

I am on treatment for high blood pressure. I know that some medications cause side effects. What should I look for?

If you feel unwell and are taking tablets, do not stop or modify your treatment in any way, but contact your doctor. He will advise what changes or modifications are necessary. This is an important point to remember because a sudden stoppage of treatment can produce what is called a 'rebound effect' in the level of blood pressure (it shoots up).

Remember that some of the symptoms given below are just as likely to be due to your blood pressure rising as to it being overtreated, i. e. there may be a need to change, reduce or increase your tablets. Therefore, if you experience:

- headaches
- visual disturbances (blurred vision)
- shortness of breath
- chest pain
- altered ability to concentrate
- memory loss
- passing more urine at night or
- sexual problems/impotence

seek your doctor's advice, but do not alter your treatment on your own.

I have heard that blood pressure pills can affect your sex life – is this true?

The short answer is sometimes. The usual complaint is of men failing to get an erection firm enough or lasting long enough for sexual intercourse. Blood pressure itself can cause this problem and only occasionally are the drugs used to treat it incriminated. If it is drug induced it will occur in the first 2–4 weeks of therapy and a different drug can then be tried. The least likely drugs to cause male erectile dysfunction (ED) are the AII antagonists (see Table 2.2) and the alpha-blockers. Female problems with lack of arousal have been reported with beta-blockers. Both men and women can get sexual problems as a result of heart disease and sometimes its treatment so, if you have a problem, talk about it with your doctor or practice nurse. There is more on this subject in Chapter 8.

While I am taking my tablets, can I lead a normal life or is there anything I should avoid doing?

Although treatment controls blood pressure effectively throughout the day, it is only sensible to avoid as much as possible any events or circumstances that increase your blood pressure, such as highly emotional or stressful situations (see section on *Stress* below)

Maintain an acceptable weight (Chapter 9), moderate your alcohol, fat and salt intake and give up cigarettes if you smoke; you should then be able to live as normal a life as possible, including a normal sex life. Above all, you should not consider yourself an invalid – you are not!

I am told that I have high blood pressure and need treatment, but I don't seem to have any symptoms. If I do not feel unwell, why should I need it?

Very often high blood pressure does not make you feel ill. This is possibly because the increase has been gradual over such a long time that you have adjusted to it. However, all the evidence shows that, if high blood pressure is left untreated, you have a greater chance of stroke, heart attacks and complications in the kidneys and eyes. When blood pressure is treated, there is overwhelming evidence that these risks are substantially reduced. Therefore, it is important, and in your interest, to take your medication exactly as prescribed by your doctor, even though you may feel quite well.

Now that I have been prescribed tablets, how long will my treatment last?

The treatment for high blood pressure, whether by lifestyle changes or drugs or both, continues for life, but as many of the medications used in its treatment need to be taken only once daily, interference with your normal lifestyle can be kept to a minimum in the majority of cases. Sometimes, if you have reached your target weight, you may have your tablets reduced or stopped, in order to see if you still need them. Ask your doctor if this is worth a try for you.

I don't mind taking one tablet a day, but one of my friends has so many that she rattles. Will these tablets be all that I need to take?

With some patients other factors or conditions may complicate the situation and treatment for these may also be required; you may then have to take several tablets a day. For example, if you develop angina, the tablets may need to be changed to relieve you of your chest pain (see the section on *Treatment* in Chapter 3). If you develop diabetes, specific diabetic tablets may be needed. We try to tailor the treatment to the individual, aiming to keep your quality of life as good as possible – so if a diuretic causes gout, we can change to a beta-blocker, and so on. We try to give you the minimum of inconvenience, but also to keep you in good health.

What should I do if I forget to take my tablets?

For most people, there is no need to worry, as the blood pressure will only rise slowly, so you can get back on schedule the next day. If you are on a beta-blocker and also have angina, you should take the medication immediately you realize that you have forgotten it, as a means of catching up.

Risks of high cholesterol levels

Facts and figures

There is a lot of talk these days about lipids and cholesterol and now I've seen something about triglycerides! I am rather muddled about it all. Can you tell me what all these words mean?

Cholesterol is a fatty or oily substance and is one of a group of fatty substances we call *lipids*.

Lipids are essential for the normal functioning of the body's cells. Problems develop when there is too much lipid in the blood. It then settles in the walls of the arteries. The arteries then develop the narrowings which cause heart attacks and angina by restricting the flow of blood to the heart (see the *Introduction* to this chapter). Doctors often ask for a 'lipid profile': this is a check on your levels of cholesterol and *triglycerides* (another fatty substance – see below).

Cholesterol plays an essential role in helping our glands make hormones, but its biggest role is in the formation of cell walls. We are able to make all the cholesterol we need in the liver, where it is made from fat. Our problems begin if we have a higher blood cholesterol than we need and this is usually due to eating too much fat (see the question later on *hypercholesterolaemia*).

Triglycerides (pronounced *try-gli-sir-ides*) are the major form of saturated fats (see later question) which come from food and they are also made in the body to provide energy. If you have a high level of triglycerides and a low level of high density lipoproteins (see next question), you have a greater chance of developing coronary disease. Triglycerides are commonly raised in people who are very overweight, people with diabetes and those who have a high alcohol intake.

I was told that all cholesterol is bad for you. Now I read that there is a 'good' cholesterol and 'bad' cholesterol. What's the difference?

Cholesterol and other fats do not dissolve in the blood. They hitch a ride on proteins which are the taxis transporting the fats around. The combination of fat and protein is a *lipoprotein* (pronounced *lie-po-pro-teen*). The 'bad' cholesterol is the *low density lipoprotein* (LDL): this is the main carrier of harmful cholesterol to your arteries where it builds up to cause narrowings. The *high density lipoproteins* (HDL) are the good guys: HDL tends to pick up excess cholesterol taking it away from the arteries and transporting it back to the liver for removal. So, you need:

- your LDL low (L for lousy)
- your HDL high (H for happy)

to give yourself maximum protection.

I'm going to have a complete check-up next month. When I have my cholesterol profile checked, what levels should all these different fats be?

Your total *cholesterol* should not be above 5.2 mmol/litre with the HDL (see question above) greater than 1.0 mmol/litre, and the LDL 3.2 mmol/litre or less (ideal 2.6 or less). Your *triglycerides* should be less than 2.0 mmol/litre (ideal 1.6 or less). As a rule of thumb a total cholesterol of 4.8 equals an LDL of 3.2. Research has shown that lowering cholesterol to these levels in normal people as well as coronary patients, helps prevent heart disease in the future. The benefits apply to both men and women.

When I had a lipid profile done on my blood, the doctor told me I had hypercholesterolaemia? What does this mean?

Hypercholesterolaemia (pronounced *hi-per-kol-esterol-eemia*) means that the total cholesterol is high in the blood. Usually the LDL (see question above) is raised; in women the HDL is higher before the menopause – an effect of their hormones. It is always better to know both profiles (HDL and LDL), as well as the total level, because you don't want to lower a high HDL by mistake. For example, a woman before the menopause may have a high total cholesterol (e. g. 5.8) which is made up mainly of the good HDL (e. g. 2.0).

When I look at a food label, there are different types of fats listed, such as saturated and unsaturated fats. Can you explain more about the differences between the types of fats?

There are two main sorts of fats.

- *Saturated fats* are mainly of animal origin. They are the bad fats and it is the saturated fat that raises your cholesterol levels.

- *Unsaturated fats* are mainly of vegetable origin and they lower your cholesterol levels.

Saturated fats are a mixture of alcohol, glycerol and fatty acids. The fatty acids contain long chains of carbon atoms – most commonly 12, 14 or 16. These are the most effective at raising the LDL ('bad cholesterol') in the blood. The more saturated fat we eat, the higher the cholesterol; if we eat less, our cholesterol will fall over 3–4 weeks.

Unsaturated fats contain carbon atoms that are joined (double bonds) at certain points; this leads to the fats being liquid or soft at room temperature. When there is one double bond, the fat is *monounsaturated*; when there are two or more, it is *polyunsaturated*. Monounsaturated fats include olive, rapeseed and peanut oils and are contained in avocados, almonds and oily fish Polyunsaturated fats include sunflower oil and most soft margarines(always read the label!). Polyunsaturated fats help prevent blood clots forming, which is another benefit in addition to their cholesterol-lowering effect.

As well as lowering your LDL (bad) cholesterol by switching you away from saturated fat, unsaturated fats also appear to have an additional good effect on lowering cholesterol. Mono-unsaturated fat may raise the HDL (good) cholesterol as well. All kinds of fat, whether saturated or unsaturated, are rich in calories, so you need to bear in mind, when you change to a healthy diet, not to go overboard on unsaturated fat.

Chapter 9 gives lots of information about which foods contain the different types of fats and gives you lists from which you can choose a healthy diet.

The media has also talked about the harmful effects of trans fatty acids. How can I avoid them?

Trans fatty acids are present in small quantities in meat and dairy products but are present in larger quantities in those oils which have been manufactured to be firmer at room temperature (i. e. when oils have been made into margarines or spreads) by a process known as *hydrogenation*. Trans fatty acids raise LDL and lower HDL cholesterol levels. When you are selecting vegetable oils and margarine it is important to look for the trans content. The best oils are blended vegetable oils, rapeseed oil and soft margarines that are low in saturates and trans fatty acids, but high in polyunsaturates and monounsaturates (see the question above). Always read the margarine label.

The article that I read also mentioned vitamin E as being beneficial. Why is it important?

Vitamin E is an *antioxidant*; antioxidants are good things to help protect the body from 'free radicals'. *Free radicals* are produced by some of the normal chemical reactions in the body cells. They are unstable and, in excess, can damage the lining of the cells by oxidizing LDL ('bad') cholesterol, causing it to stick to the walls of the arteries.

Antioxidants are present in fruit and vegetables and can prevent cholesterol being oxidized so that it does not tend to stick to the artery wall. Some early studies suggested that vitamin E protects against heart disease, but unfortunately subsequent studies have not shown any benefit from tablet supplements. Vitamin E is present in food containing a lot of polyunsaturates, such as vegetable oils (especially sunflower) and deep green leafy vegetables. Nuts and vegetable oils, although good sources of vitamin E, are also high in calories, so these should not be eaten too frequently. There is a small amount of vitamin E in wholemeal bread. Some margarines are enriched with vitamin E. If your food intake is high in polyunsaturates, it will contain a lot of vitamin E. Because some of the major sources are high in calories, you may be advised to take extra vitamin E as supplementary tablets by some specialists to avoid putting on weight, but for most of us this will not be necessary. Chemists and health food shops sell vitamin E preparations and the recommended dose is 100–200 units a day (70–140 mg). However, as vitamin supplements have been shown to be of no benefit – save your money!

You have talked about vitamin E. What about vitamin C – isn't this an antioxidant as well?

Yes, and it is safe to take, but medical trials have demonstrated no benefit for heart disease. It is found in citrus fruits (oranges, grapefruits, lemons etc.), kiwi fruit, soft fruit (strawberries, raspberries, blackberries etc.), red and green peppers and spring greens. Try to eat 150–200 g (6–8 oz) of this group a day and you will not need tablet supplements.

I have always believed taking vitamin supplements would protect me – are you saying this is not true?

Unfortunately yes. The Heart Protection Study involved thousands of patients and those taking vitamins did no better or worse than those taking *placebos* (fakes). In other words, vitamins do not protect against the effects of hardening of the arteries and are of no benefit to the heart. The vitamin story is a good example of an idea that is theoretically good but, when tested, does not work.

I know of people taking beta carotene supplements and our health food shop is always marketing it – should I be taking them, and what is beta carotene?

No. Beta carotene is converted in the body to vitamin A. It is an antioxidant and is found in brightly coloured fruit and vegetables (carrots, broccoli, tomatoes, melons, yellow and orange peppers, spinach, peaches). So you might think that extra supplements would be good for you. However, medical trials have failed to show that they have any benefit, and researchers are now worried that they may lead to an increased risk of some cancers and heart disease. Do not waste your money on beta carotene supplements – fruit and vegetables are all that you need.

I thought that people supplementing their diet with extra beta carotene from the health food shops had a lower chance of developing heart disease or cancer. You say that there may be risk of developing these conditions – which view is right?

This question is a good example of the need to make sure always that a good idea works when put into practice. Beta carotene has antioxidant properties and, in theory, could help prevent cancer and coronary heart disease. Indeed, people who took beta carotene supplements were *observed* to be less likely to develop these diseases – but an observation is not proof. Four research studies involving thousands of people set out to prove whether a benefit existed when beta carotene was compared to placebo (see the section on *Other treatments for angina* in Chapter 3). These were proper scientific studies. Surprisingly and alarmingly, beta carotene supplements were shown to *increase* heart disease and cancer risks, especially in smokers and people exposed to asbestos. Ideas, whether based on good scientific theory as in the case of beta carotene or dreamed up in the bath, should always be validated! Beta carotene should be consumed normally in fresh fruit and vegetables.

There is so much advice about fat intake that I really don't know what to believe. How much fat should we eat a day?

This depends on whether you need to reduce weight, i. e. reduce calories. Remember that fat, whether good (unsaturated) or bad (saturated) is high in calories. We need 50–90 g of fat a day of which 22–27 g, only, should be saturates. Always look on the food labels to help you choose foods that contain less saturated fats.

First let's work out some numbers. Doctors recommend 30% of your calorie intake as fat, and 10% as saturated fat, and this is regardless of whether or not you are overweight. If your daily calorie intake is 1500 kcal, this means 50 g of fat at most (1 g of fat equals 9 kcal); if it is 2000 kcal, this means 65–70 g of fat; if it is 2500 kcal, this means 85-90 g of fat. (See Chapter 9 for further information on fats in food.)

My father had a high cholesterol level and died aged 55. My wife is concerned that I may be like him – I am now 52. Can this be inherited?

Some people may inherit a high cholesterol level (usually over 8.0 mmol/litre). A good diet changes these people's levels only marginally and they will need medication. Make sure that all members of your family are checked for an inherited pattern and, if this is detected, you will be recommended medication. Other people inherit a tendency to a high cholesterol level but respond to diet or, more usually, a combination of diet and medications.

Self-help

Should I know my cholesterol and other test level numbers? Will it do any good?

If you want to reduce your chances of heart disease, you must take charge of your lifestyle, and that includes knowing your numbers and keeping track of how they respond to any changes in your eating pattern or medication.

How well will a healthy diet lower my cholesterol?

A healthy diet may reduce your cholesterol by 10%. Obviously the higher your cholesterol at the start, the more likely you will need medications as well, but a period of healthy diet restricting your fat intake for 3 months is normally recommended first (see Chapter 9). However, if you already have heart problems, most doctors advise immediate medication to take full advantage of its cholesterol-lowering effect.

Which is more important – to avoid foods high in cholesterol or saturated fats?

Cholesterol in your food has a smaller effect on the blood cholesterol level than do foods high in saturated fat. It is more important therefore to cut down on foods high in saturated fat. This means, for example, that you can have three to four eggs a week (the yolks are high in cholesterol). Cutting down on saturated fat (and all fats) will help you to lose weight (see Chapter 9).

I am told that I have a high cholesterol level. If I manage to lower this level, will this really prevent heart disease?

We now have overwhelming evidence that lowering your cholesterol level not only reduces your risks of heart disease by an average of over 30%, but also reduces the need for heart bypass surgery and angioplasty (see Chapter 3). If you lower your cholesterol over a 5-year period, you improve your chances of living longer by an amazing 30%. Treating a high cholesterol is one of the most important means of preventing and reducing the complications of coronary artery disease. Some doctors believe it is negligent not to lower a raised cholesterol.

What should I get my cholesterol levels down to in order to see a benefit to my heart?

Most of the benefit occurs when the LDL ('bad') cholesterol is lowered by 30% or more; your aim should be to get this level below 3.2 mmol/litre with an ideal of 2.6 mmol/litre or less. This leads to removal of the soft part of the narrowings in the arteries making them less likely to tear or split. It is known as stabilizing the plaque (see the *Introduction* to this chapter). Unstable plaque that ruptures releases soft cholesterol into the blood which then causes a clot to form and a possible heart attack to occur – removing the soft cholesterol helps to prevent this happening.

I have reduced my cholesterol level so that the tests are now normal. Can I go back to smoking?

No. Risk factors, which increase your chances of developing heart problems, are independent of each other. If you have more than one risk factor, however, they don't just add up, they multiply.

I have seen self-testing kits for cholesterol in the chemists. Are these any good?

Not really. They are not as accurate as we had hoped they would be.

Do I need to starve for the blood test?

A blood sample which will show the levels for total cholesterol and HDL can be taken at any time. and this will be a useful screening test. However, the LDL and triglyceride levels are influenced by diet and should be measured after at least nine hours of fasting.

My doctor has only measured my total cholesterol level. Is this enough, or should I ask for all the different levels to be measured?

When your doctor is giving you a screening test, the total cholesterol level is a good guide. A total cholesterol of 5.2 or less is satisfactory and remember that 4.8 of total cholesterol is equal to 3.2 of 'bad' LDL. However, if your doctor is planning your treatment, a full lipid profile is needed to guide therapy properly. If you are going to be on medication for a long time, you need to be sure that you are on the right type.

When should I have a repeat cholesterol level test?

When you have been on your new healthy diet for 3 months, the doctor will ask you to come in for another test.

Treatment

What happens if my second cholesterol level test is still raised?

You will need medication. Fortunately the medications that you might be given are safe, simple to use and very effective – usually your cholesterol levels will begin to fall within 21 days.

What medications are there to treat high cholesterol levels and are there any side effects?

The commonest medications that you may be prescribed are known as the statins (Table 2.4). They reduce the production of cholesterol in the liver. Side effects are rare but you may get indigestion, muscle aches and pains, an itchy rash, sleep disturbance and possibly a reduced sex drive or impotence. After you have been on one of these medications for 3–4 weeks, your doctor will want to check your cholesterol again to make sure that the dose is right and that you are not suffering from any of these side effects. Always tell your doctor if you feel that you are having side effects.

The next most common group of medications is the fibrates. These are used more when your HDL is low and your triglycerides high. Stomach upsets occur sometimes as a side effect.

Sachets of medications known as the resins are used less these days as they can cause a lot of stomach troubles and they taste like sand.

A combination of medications is occasionally used to increase their effect, when a single medication is not enough to get the levels right.

Table 2.4 Cholesterol-lowering drugs

Drugs	Effects	Side effects
Statins Atorvastatin (Lipitor)	Lower LDL by over 20% and up to 50%	Rare stomach upsets; muscle pains; sleep disturbance
Fluvastatin (Lescol) Pravastatin (Lipostat) Simvastatin (Zocor) Rosuvastatin (Crestor)		
Fibrates Fenofibrate (Lipantil)	Raise HDL, lower triglycerides (30%)	Uncommon stomach upsets; muscle pains
Ciprofibrate (Modalim) Bezafibrate (Bezalip) Gemfibrozil (Lopid)		
Resins Cholestyramine (Questran)	Lower LDL but raise triglycerides	Constipation; bloating, gas

I have been prescribed cholesterol-lowering medication, although I am only 50. Will I always need medication?

Usually yes. Occasionally, after a time when you have been losing weight and eating healthily, the medication can be stopped for a month to see what happens; usually your cholesterol goes up again, but at least you've proved that you *do* need medication.

If you have coronary disease, lowering your cholesterol will help reduce your chances of a heart attack or the need for heart surgery or angioplasty. Lowering your cholesterol will also help to lengthen your life. For most people, one or, occasionally, two tablets a day plus a healthy lifestyle are all that is needed. The tablets are easy to take with few side effects. This is one occasion when 'keep on taking the tablets' is very good advice and, in terms of health care, very good value.

When I have finally got my cholesterol level under control, how often should I have it checked?

Every 12 months.

I have been on cholesterol-lowering medication for some time now. When I go for a check-up, my doctor checks my liver. Why?

It is in the liver that the statins, in particular, get to work, and, very rarely, cause an upset; the tablets then have to be stopped. If you are unfortunate enough to have this side effect, you will be pleased to know that the liver will get better, once the medication has been withdrawn.

Can lowering cholesterol levels be harmful, as I have read that lowering cholesterol increases the chances of suffering a violent death or suicide?

There were some reports suggesting this but, by proper scientific study, they have been disproved. This is called evidence-based medicine. Lowering cholesterol reduces your chance of dying from heart disease and doe *not* increase your chance of dying from anything else.

I have had a heart attack and even though my cholesterol was only 4.5 I have been put on a statin – why is this?

If you have coronary disease, the level of cholesterol at which you developed it is too high for you. Studies have shown a significant benefit in reducing heart attacks, strokes or death in those with known coronary disease or those at high risk (e.g. those with diabetes), who start with a cholesterol as low as 3.5 mmol/litre. Statins have other properties other than lowering cholesterol and can reduce the inflammation in the narrowing of arteries, preventing disruption. So, once the disease is known about, the treatment is more aggressive because the benefits are substantial.

I have read about a new cholesterol drug called Ezetrol – when is this used?

Ezetrol is the trade name for ezetimibe a drug that acts to prevent the absorption of cholesterol in the bowel. It is a fixed dose of 10 mg and lowers LDL cholesterol by 10–20% when acting on its own or added to statin therapy. Side effects are not common – mainly nausea and bloating and in only 2% of people taking it. It is used when statins are not tolerated at all or when the dose needed to achieve your target for LDL cholesterol causes side effects – it can then be added to a lower dose of statin, which is tolerated, to get an additive effect.

Other risk factors for coronary heart disease

Being overweight – obesity

I don't feel overweight but the doctor says I am. Have I got more chance of developing heart disease because of this?

Very overweight (*obese*) people do have more chance of developing heart disease and this has been mentioned earlier (see section on **Risks of high blood pressure**). Being fat increases the work the heart has to do, causes high blood pressure and leads to abnormal blood lipids (*hypercholesterolaemia*). It can also lead to you developing diabetes (see below). You should try to reduce your weight – see Chapter 9 for advice about healthy eating and losing weight. Big bellies are bad for your heart!

Stress

I have a very stressful job. Am I more likely to get heart problems?

There is no proof that stress actually causes heart disease but it can contribute to the symptoms. It is like a trigger, setting things off.

Stress is a state of mind not an illness so it is difficult to obtain a precise measurement of it. We all feel stress but it affects us in different ways and we respond differently. Under stress people may smoke or drink more, overeat for comfort or have slightly higher blood pressures.

Stress can be fun as well as unpleasant, for example watching a close team match or taking part yourself in team games. A sudden acute stressful incident is the most dangerous (such as a near-miss on the motorway) but usually cannot be avoided. Stress interacts with your chances of developing heart disease and can make them worse.

Will I be able to recognize the symptoms of dangerous levels of stress?

Symptoms will vary but, in general, when stress is detrimental, you will become tense, nervous and often afraid; you may sleep badly, wake early and have tension pains in the muscles of the neck or back.

Is there any way I can reduce my stress levels?

Yes, there are various ways you can help yourself.

- Try to remove yourself from a stressful environment for some of the day. If work is stressful, go for a walk at lunch-time. Keep physically active.

- Don't rely on caffeine or alcohol and don't smoke.

- Learn that you alone cannot solve all life's problems and that they are not all caused by you.

- Try relaxation tapes, yoga or deep breathing exercises. These work well for some people (see below).

- Spend less time with people who irritate you.

- Try to avoid rush-hour travel (leave for work earlier and walk the last mile or so).

- Talk through any problems at work or with friends (don't repress them and let them fester).

- Avoid overcommitment – be positive but don't be afraid to turn things down.

- Don't rush about, take your time, plan what you are going to do and follow it through – again be positive and don't be deflected.

- Most of all, keep life in perspective – yesterday is gone, tomorrow hasn't happened, just get on with today and enjoy it.

The most important therapy is your own. Look at what you are doing and ask what your priorities are. If you had one day left in your life, would you shout and yell in traffic, or swear at the railway guard because the train is late (again!), or would you spend time with your loved ones, telling them how much they mean to you. Take deep breaths and keep the world in proportion. If you must do something, punch a pillow but laugh at yourself as you do it!

Really stressed people usually have other psychological problems which benefit from counselling or a support group. If you are unlucky enough to have a heart attack, a 'cardiac rehabilitation programme' is invariably helpful. It provides expert help and support as well as guidance on exercise and a healthy lifestyle. It is usually run by nurses who understand your fears and worries, and can help you regain your confidence.

Diffuse your feelings by using art, music, dance and exercise as a relief valve. There are many videos, tapes and books on stress management which people have found useful. Any relaxation technique will help. Yoga is a very useful exercise and is an ideal way to wind down and relax. Take evening classes which will allow you to meet others and get away from your normal daily routine.

Above all else, remember that by bringing stress under control you will not only benefit your heart but also improve your outlook on life, allowing better and more complete relationships with loved ones, friends and colleagues at work.

Why is so much emphasis placed on stress in the media?

This is a lot of money in stress management and it is an easy diagnostic dustbin. If you have a funny illness, it is 'a virus'; if you can't explain something, it is 'stress'!

I have read about type 'A' and 'B' personalities having an effect on the heart. What is the difference between them?

Some psychiatrists divide the world into two groups, type A and type B people. Type A people are competitive, intense and driven by success. Type B are relaxed, unhurried and content with their lives and achievements. Type A personality has been linked to heart disease but several studies have failed to establish a direct connection. It may well be the consequences of a type A personality that establish a relationship with heart problems, reflecting the degree of anger and frustration that these people feel rather than their attitudes and activities alone.

Do different emotions affect the heart adversely?

Anger appears to be the most dangerous emotion, increasing heart strain by raising blood pressure and increasing heart rate. If you are angry, write a letter about the person or problem, expressing your anger, then tear it up. (Don't send it!) Yell and shout at a mirror, then laugh at yourself as you regain perspective. Learn to count to 10 slowly, while breathing deeply.

I feel that I am stressed at the end of the day. What can I do?

You are probably overdoing things and overcommitted. Look at your day: can you organize it better?

- Does anyone or any issue stress you more? If so, bring it into the open.
- Walk some of the way to work and try to get out at lunch-time.
- If you feel trapped in your home all day, make the effort to go out – go window shopping, walk round a shopping mall if it is raining; walk in the park if it's fine.
- Complete the day with deep breathing exercises, have a warm soak in the bath, clean your teeth and freshen up.

- Read a book, do a crossword, work on a hobby project, or 'surf the net' and think about your priorities.

- If you have a pet, pat it or stroke it – play with the cat, or walk the dog.

Stress is usually present when emotions are bottled up and everything gets out of perspective.

Diabetes

I have had diabetes for 30 years. What is the effect of diabetes on heart disease?

People with diabetes do have more heart disease than those without. Whilst very good and strict sugar control may reduce some of the risk, this is undone by an increased number of hypoglycaemic attacks. Although you can't help having diabetes and, unfortunately, it cannot yet be cured, you can help the other factors that cause heart disease. Do not smoke, keep as fit as you can and avoid getting overweight; keep your cholesterol in check and aim for a normal blood pressure.

Many doctors put diabetics routinely on statins to reduce the risk no matter what the cholesterol is.

I have diabetes and have now been told that I have insulin resistance and am at risk of heart disease – what is insulin resistance?

Normally, when you eat food, your blood sugar (glucose) levels go up; your body produces insulin as a response; insulin helps glucose to be taken up by the tissues, the glucose in your blood falls, and then your insulin level falls. It is called a negative feedback mechanism. If you are insulin-resistant the action of insulin in the tissues is less effective than it should be and glucose (sugar) is not used properly, so the sugar and insulin levels remain raised because the feedback is interrupted. Insulin in high levels can raise the blood pressure, cause salt and water retention and raise LDL ('bad') cholesterol and lower HDL ('good') cholesterol. Therefore, yes, insulin resistance can increase your risks of developing heart disease.

Being overweight, particularly abdominal obesity (a fat belly), is associated with or causes insulin resistance and Type 2 diabetes. By reducing weight both diabetes and insulin resistance can be controlled or even overcome. It is more common among Indo-Asian people. Besides reducing your weight, you can also take medications to lower insulin resistance including the ACE inhibitors (see the section ***Risks of high blood pressure*** earlier in this chapter).

Illegal drugs

I worry that my teenage daughter might have access to drugs. Do illegal drugs affect young people's chances of heart problems?

Cannabis (or 'pot' or marijuana) increases the heart rate and blood pressure as well as body temperature. It also contains carbon monoxide in the smoke. Although it can help some medical problems, e. g. the nausea of cancer therapy, severe pain

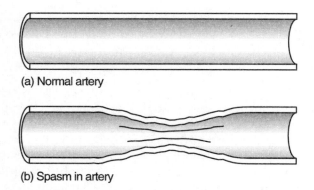

(a) Normal artery

(b) Spasm in artery

Figure 2.6 Lengthways section of (**a**) a normal artery and (**b**) an artery in spasm, which narrows the opening available for blood flow.

and multiple sclerosis, heart problems is not one of them and it is therefore not recommended.

Cocaine ('crack') is a powerful addictive drug which can cause blood vessels to shut down (go into spasm) (Figure 2.6). It can raise blood pressure, cause strokes and lead to severe heart disease, provoking irregular heart beats, inflaming heart muscle and causing heart attacks. Just one 'fix' can do it – my advice is don't try it.

You may have heard that *morphine* helps the heart. It is not that simple. Children may begin with the idea of taking heroin (related to morphine) in small amounts and keeping it under control, but the addiction takes over, infection risks rise (from dirty needles or impure products), the heart valves can become severely damaged and the heart, overwhelmed by disease, gives up functioning properly. This leads to heart failure, resulting in a rapid and inevitable premature death.

If you think your child may be addicted, seek help. Help is available for recovery but an addict needs to admit to addiction, want to end it and accept help from professionals.

Ecstasy has been very much in the news. Taking even one ecstasy tablet is akin to committing suicide. It may cause a very high fever, irreversible brain damage and heart failure.

Women and coronary heart disease

I am a mother aged 53. I am concerned to read that coronary heart disease is a major risk for me. I thought it was a man's disease.

Of the deaths from heart attacks each year, nearly half are in women. All forms of heart and blood vessel diseases added together claim twice as many women's lives as do all forms of cancer. Although fewer women have heart disease than men at the age of 50, they have caught up by 65–70 years of age. The main difference between men and women as regards heart disease is not *if* they are going to get coronary disease, but *when*; the difference in its timing is about 10 years.

Coronary heart disease is therefore your – and other women's – biggest problem too. It is becoming more of a woman's disease as women tend to live longer; coronary disease is partly a problem of getting older, so more women will eventually develop it. The problem is going to increase as the population ages in general. More men and women are now surviving heart attacks, so they are likely to encounter heart problems later – an increased chance of angina or a further heart attack, unless they try to reduce their risks. Women are more vulnerable to the risks of cigarette smoking and high blood pressure but less so to that of cholesterol. Having diabetes sadly wipes out any advantages that women may have had over men (see above).

My father had heart disease and I am concerned that my daughter might develop heart disease also. I know that she smokes. How can I help her avoid heart disease?

Your daughter may have an increased risk of heart disease if it runs in your family but one of the best ways to help prevent coronary heart disease is to get her to stop smoking. It is well known that there has been an increase in the numbers of young women smoking; their chances of heart disease in later life consequently are rising. If your daughter smokes, she should stop now. If she is thinking about starting -, she should think again!

I have read that women's natural hormones protect us from heart disease. Is this true?

To a degree they do, but if you smoke, have high blood pressure or have diabetes, women lose a lot of this protection. Following the menopause, the normal protection that oestrogen gives disappears anyway, Hormone replacement therapy (HRT) (see below) unfortunately does not appear to help.

I have been taking the pill on and off since I was 18. I have just been through the menopause. Am I at any greater risk of heart disease because I have been using oral contraceptives?

Very few women on the pill (taking oral contraceptives) develop heart disease and the low hormone dose pills do not increase the coronary risk. So long as you do not smoke, the low dose pill may actually protect you against heart problems. In women under 35 years of age we do not know what the risk is from taking the pill, nor do we know about its long-term use (over 5 years), although it is unlikely you will be harmed. Cigarette smoking and also taking the pill is not a good combination and should be avoided at all costs. In general the low dose pills are safe, but smokers should preferably stop smoking, or use alternative contraception.

I have felt well since being on HRT but I am worried about its affect on my heart and the risk of breast cancer – what should I do?

There is no doubt that HRT helps with the distressing symptoms of menopausal flushes and protects against thinning of the bones (osteoporosis). Initial enthusiasm regarding HRT and heart disease has been replaced with sound scientific evidence of a *lack* of benefit. Currently HRT is not recommended as a treatment to prevent heart disease developing or to benefit women who have heart disease already. If coronary disease has been diagnosed, other protective treatments should be used – for example statin therapy. Some studies have suggested HRT can actually increase the risk of heart disease, but this risk does not appear to be present if the cholesterol is normal or a statin is also being taken.

A very big study – The Million Women Study – has identified an increased risk of breast cancer if the HRT is taken for 5 years or more. We are looking at 1 extra case of breast cancer in 166 women treated for 5 years or 1 extra case in 53 women treated for 10 years. There is no need to panic about these figures, but clearly women on HRT for many years should see their family doctor about discontinuing.

The HRT story is a sad journey from the belief of benefit to the proof of potential harm. There is no role for HRT in women who do not have menopausal symptoms (flushes, etc.). When flushes are a problem (this happens in 10–20% of women), the risks must be weighed against the benefit, and HRT used for as short a time as possible.

Most women are on combined medications of oestrogen and progestogen but, if they have had a hysterectomy (womb removed), they will be on oestrogen alone. All increase the breast cancer risk. With regard to the heart, we are not sure about oestrogen alone but, with all the information we have, HRT cannot be considered a treatment for heart disease.

Whether this advice will change when we know more about raloxifene (see next question) is debateable, but it is obviously important to continue research in this area and advise women on up-to-date scientific facts.

I have read in the paper about a new drug called raloxifene – what advantage dose this have?

Raloxifene is one of a class of drugs called Selective Estrogen (American spelling) Receptor Modulators or SERMS. Tamoxifen is the one we already have but tamoxifen can sometimes, as a side effect, cause the uterus (womb) lining to overgrow and become troublesome. Raloxifene acts the same as tamoxifen in benefiting the heart and bones, avoids breast cancer risks and does not affect the womb. It is an important drug but like tamoxifen does not reduce hot flushes. It may be an important advance in HRT for women because it looks to have the major benefits without the major risks. A lot of research is taking place to determine how valuable it will be to the heart – proof is not yet available, but early results do not show any harm.

Does HRT have any side effects?

All medication can give side effects and HRT is no exception. You may feel nauseous but it usually goes after 2 weeks or so – taking tablets after a meal can help this. Breast tenderness and swelling may occur and, again, wear off but, if persistent, you may be given a different form of HRT to try.

Women worry about gaining weight whilst on HRT. The many research trials do not report weight gain but you should remember that everyone is an individual and if you gain weight, it is you that matters, not the statistics. It is probably due to eating more as you feel better on HRT! Watching your weight is important anyway, so at this time take note of what you are eating and make sure that you take plenty of exercise.

On average, women take 3 months to settle into their HRT therapy.

Does HRT raise blood pressure?

Very rarely. Your doctor or nurse will always check your blood pressure when HRT is prescribed. If you have high blood pressure, you can still take HRT because the chances of your control being upset are so small, and this risk is dwarfed by the benefits in lowering your chance of heart disease.

I have breast cancer which is now controlled, and I have also had a heart attack – will HRT help me?

It will not obviously help the heart and it could make the breast cancer worse, so it is not recommended. HRT is not an alternative to proven heart attack treatments.

What sort of HRT therapy is available?

The choice of therapy is best discussed with your doctor. There are two sorts: the first is oestrogen only and this type is for women who have had a hysterectomy (removal of the womb) – this is known as 'unopposed oestrogen'. The second type is 'combined' HRT (containing oestrogen and progesterone) for women who still have a womb, because oestrogen alone in these women will cause excess stimulation of the lining of the womb.

I have been advised to go on HRT but I am resisting as I have read that it doubles your chances of getting blood clots in the legs – is this true?

Yes this is true. Your normal risk of getting a dangerous blood clot is 1 in 10 000 and it increases to 2 in 10 000 on HRT. So the risk is very small and remains very small on HRT. The risk is higher in those over 60 years of age, but HRT is rarely started in this age group. Talk to your doctor about this, if you think that you may be at risk.

I'm fit and active with no risk factors for heart disease – will I benefit from HRT?

If you have no risks for heart disease, HRT will not improve this as your risk is very low anyway, but you may benefit from HRT by avoiding osteoporosis (thin bones). This is more common in slim women. HRT also helps to relieve hot flushes. Check with your doctor about the possibility of having a bone density scan if you think you may be at risk for osteoporosis.

From the point of view of heart health, who will benefit most from taking HRT?

No one.

I have been taking HRT for 7 years and I think that it is wonderful – I now feel a new woman! However, my doctor says that I should stop it soon. How long should I continue taking HRT?

HRT is usually taken for hot flushes for up to 5 years. Bone benefits continue on beyond 10 years, but the breast cancer risk increases. So, at present, we recommend HRT is stopped.

I'm on HRT at the moment. Do I need regular check-ups?

It is very important that you attend for regular check-ups at first every 3 months and then 6 monthly, and follow your doctor's instructions. For these check-ups, make a note of any queries or concerns that you might have and discuss them with your doctor.

I have been on oral HRT for some months and my doctor has arranged for me to have a lipid test. Why?

The doctor is checking to make sure that you are not at risk, which is good medical practice. Up to the menopause, women usually have a raised high density lipoprotein level (HDL) (greater than 1.3) which helps protect them from coronary disease. This HDL gradually falls after the menopause unless HRT is taken. It is important that women should always have a full lipid profile taken (HDL as well as LDL) because a high total cholesterol may reflect good (HDL) rather than bad (LDL) cholesterol levels. Reducing your total cholesterol in this situation might reduce the protective HDL and be counter-productive.

A full lipid profile will also tell you about your triglycerides. Oral HRT can raise triglycerides, but HRT patches have no effect on triglyceride levels. A high triglyceride level is more of a risk in women than in men and the best means of lowering it is by weight loss and regular exercise, along with a low saturated fat diet. An underactive thyroid and too much alcohol can also be a cause.

I do find the advice on HRT confusing – can you clarify it for me?

I'll try, but doctors find it confusing too!

- HRT definitely helps menopausal symptoms, such as hot flushes.
- It definitely helps prevent thin bones (osteoporosis).
- It does not protect against heart disease developing.

- In those with coronary disease, it does not benefit them, so it is not a treatment for heart disease.
- In those with heart disease, it still helps menopausal symptoms and osteoporosis.
- HRT increases the risk of breast cancer.
- Overall, HRT is indicated only if menopausal symptoms are severe and intolerable, and is given for as short a time as possible.

I'm concerned that my wife is at risk of heart disease and I want her to take it seriously; she smokes and is rather well padded! However, my doctor does not seem to be bothering either. What should I tell her?

You should point out that women are just as vulnerable to coronary disease as men. Some women don't recognize this and play down any symptoms of chest discomfort. They usually put their family first. Sometimes they might hide things from the doctor, which makes diagnosis difficult for both angina and a heart attack.

Your wife and every other woman should take heart disease seriously and your doctor, like all doctors, should recognize that women with a mixture of symptoms need taking seriously. Women may be reassured too easily because most women believe themselves to be less likely to have heart disease than men.

Postmenopausal women are at more risk and, even when the symptoms are not typical, these should be discussed and heart disease ruled in or out.

Women are just as likely as men to develop coronary disease if they smoke and just as likely to benefit if they stop. Keeping to a sensible weight and taking regular exercise are also important preventative measures. Tell her that heart disease is an equal opportunity killer and that she should do her best to avoid it for her sake and that of her family.

Send for the British Heart Foundation's booklet *Women and heart disease* and present it to her!

3
Angina

Each year in the UK around 320 000 people visit their doctor for angina. Over six million people in America and two million in the UK are affected. *Angina* (pronounced *ann-jy-na*) is a symptom of a problem not a disease in itself. It is usually caused by narrowing of the coronary arteries by atheroma (see introduction to Chapter 2). It can also be caused by a high blood pressure (see section on ***Risks of high blood pressure*** in Chapter 2), disease of the aortic valve (see Chapter 7), severe anaemia, and rapid palpitations (see Chapter 6) or a mixture of conditions. Far and away the commonest cause is coronary artery disease (see Chapter 2). The coronary arteries supply oxygen to the heart and the heart gets this supply between its beats, when it is refuelling itself. This means that the faster your heart beats, the less oxygen there is for the heart itself. If your arteries are narrowed, the flow is restricted. The balance will be OK when you are not doing anything but, when your heart speeds up, there will come a point when the narrow arteries restrict the supply of oxygen to your heart muscle and pain develops. This is when angina is most often felt, as a chest pain, when you are active or when you are worked up about something, because the demands of your heart for oxygen are not being met by the supply of oxygenated blood to your heart muscle.

Symptoms

My husband has got angina. He is obviously in pain but cannot describe it easily. What does it feel like?

The pain usually begins behind the breast bone. It is often felt as a tightness or a squeezing sensation; your husband probably describes it best by clenching his fist in front of his chest (Figure 3.1).

The pain of angina can be regarded as a built-in warning device and tells him that the heart has reached its maximum workload. The onset of pain or discomfort indicates that he should slow down or stop any exertion. Alternatively, if emotion (such as anger) has lead to this, then he should relax and remove himself from the situation.

Angina pain *cannot* usually be localized by pointing; it is more widespread and felt across the chest. It is brought on usually by effort, so it will build up if that effort is continued. When it begins, it is often quite mild – more of an ache – so it is easily confused with indigestion. Angina pain may spread (radiate) to the throat or neck, the jaw (like toothache), to the left or right arm or both, and sometimes to the back or stomach. It usually goes down the inside of the arm, in contrast to muscle pain which runs over the shoulder and down the outside of the arm. Rarely, angina occurs in one of these places without being in the chest, e. g. a person gets pain in the left arm on effort which is relieved by resting.

Figure 3.1 Hand movements and chest pain. Heart pain is usually described with the flat of the hand (**a**) or a clenched fist (**b**). Heart pain is almost never localized or pointed to(**c**).

Can he get chest pain from causes other than heart disease?

There are many other causes of chest pain and here are some pointers to stop you worrying unnecessarily:

- *Joint or muscle pain.* This is often worse when someone is changing position. This sort of pain can be reproduced by pressing on the ribs or breastbone.

- *Lung disorders.* This pain is aggravated when you take a deep breath.

- *Stomach problems.* Indigestion after a meal or on bending with an acid taste in your mouth (acid reflux).

- *Gallbladder problems.* Colicky pain after a fatty meal may suggest gallstones.

- *Stress, anxiety* or *overbreathing.*

Nobody should have chest pain that is a mystery. Do not assume your husband has angina but also do not let him ignore the pain. Get him to ask his doctor's advice.

What is the difference between angina and a heart attack?

Angina is the result of a temporary shortage of oxygen available to the heart muscle, usually caused by exercise or strong feelings. Angina pain usually passes off when you stop activity, or very shortly after taking a 'nitrate' tablet (see section on *Treatment* below). Angina results from narrowed coronary arteries.

A heart attack is different (see Chapter 4). The pain build-up is more severe, lasts longer and does not decrease when you stop any activity. It may be modified if you take nitrate tablets but is not relieved. You will often find that you sweat and you may feel sick. A heart attack is caused by an artery blocking off, usually when a clot forms on a narrowed area.

See Table 3.1 for the main differences in signs between angina and a heart attack.

Table 3.1 Chest pain characteristics

Typical angina pain	Not heart pain
Tightness	Sharp (not severe)
Pressure	Knife-like
Weight on the chest	Stabbing
Heaviness	'Like a stitch'
Constriction – like a band	Shooting
Ache	Localized
Dull	Positional
Burning	Reproduced by pressure
Crushing	Located elsewhere than mid-chest
Retrosternal (behind breast bone)	Not exertional
Precipitated by exercise and/or emotion	Not relieved by GTN
Relieved by antacids	
Relieved promptly by GTN*	

*GTN, glyceryl trinitrate (see section on *Medication* later in this chapter)

I have been diagnosed as having unstable angina. What is this?

Angina that occurs more frequently with ever decreasing activity (e.g. 22 metres [25 yards] walking rather than 0.8 km [half a mile]) is known as unstable angina. It may also occur at minimal activity or at rest, or wake you from sleep.

You should see your doctor urgently if:

- you are getting angina for the first time;

- the pain is getting worse and occurring more frequently;

- the pain happens when you are not doing anything.

I am on medicine for angina and I still often get pains. If I get an attack of angina, it is difficult to know when I should bother the doctor. What should I do?

There are various instances when this would be advisable:

- if you have been newly diagnosed with angina and pain occurs when you are walking less than 22 metres (25 yards) on the flat;

- if it occurs at rest (usually in bed);

- if the pain lasts longer than 20 minutes in spite of nitrates (see below);

- if you are very breathless;

- if you feel faint or light-headed with the pain;

- if the pain comes on while you are convalescing from a recent heart attack.

When should I dial 999 rather than just call a doctor?

If the pain last longer than 20 minutes, in spite of nitrate tablets or spray, then dial 999. Tell them that you need an ambulance and have a 'possible heart attack'. Try another nitrate tablet or spray if the pain continues; crunch a 300 mg tablet of aspirin and then swallow it. Aspirin thins the blood and can help prevent unstable angina developing into a heart attack as well as limiting the damage a heart attack can do.

I have angina, but I want to live an active life. Is there any activity that is likely to bring my angina on?

Any form of exercise can bring angina on – climbing stairs, carrying shopping, walking up an incline and rushing. Angina may be more of a problem in cold or windy weather, or when you are carrying something heavy or going for a walk too soon after a large meal. It also occurs when you are under emotional stress, especially anger. It can vary a lot from day to day, but if it is becoming more frequent and the distances you can walk shorter, you should report back to your doctor.

I sometimes get a pain after eating. The doctor told me this was 'postprandial angina'. What exactly is this?

As your doctor says, this is angina which occurs after a meal. Eating a large meal can increase the work that the heart has to do by 20% (to digest the food) so angina may occur if you have coronary narrowings. The usual sequence goes something like this: meal – walk the dog – angina. This happens because you have exercised too soon after a meal adding stress to the heart. Postprandial angina can be a warning of more severe coronary disease and I expect your doctor will be giving you some more tests.

Sometimes when I drive, for instance in the rush hour, I get angina symptoms – am I wise to carry on?

No. You must not drive until your symptoms are controlled, either by medication or surgery.

Tests

What tests might I have to undergo for angina?

Your doctor will examine you, check your weight and blood pressure and listen to your heart for certain sounds and noises in your chest. Your blood should be checked when you have not eaten overnight to measure the fat content (cholesterol – see the section on *Risks of high cholesterol levels* in Chapter 2).

Your doctor may want to do an *electrocardiogram* (ECG) (see below) which is a means of checking the way the heart works and whether there is any damage. An exercise electrocardiogram on a treadmill machine or bicycle may be used to assess how well your heart behaves under stress and how much you can do.

Some people may be sent to a specialist heart doctor (a cardiologist) who may suggest that you have an *angiogram*, with a cardiac catheter inserted (see the section on *Angiogram* below).

ECG

**My doctor is sending me for an ECG next week. I am not
sure what this involves – will it mean time in hospital for
an operation?**

No, and it is painless and takes only 10 minutes to do. An
electrocardiogram (ECG in the UK, EKG in Europe or the USA) is
a simple painless test which looks at the electrical activity of the
heart. It tells the doctor about your heart rate, whether you are
likely to have a heart attack and if you have any hardening of
your arteries, and whether your heart's rhythm is regular or not.

You will have electrodes (usually sticky pads) applied to your
arms and legs, and six are placed across your chest (Figure 3.2)
to record the electrical activity in your heart, while you are not
doing anything. Men with hairy chests may need a small area

Figure 3.2 An electrocardiogram is being taken while the patient is at rest.
The trace from the machine is also shown.

Figure 3.3 An electrocardiogram is being taken while the patient
is on a treadmill.

shaved. The resulting ECG trace gives an electrical picture of
your heart. It is not dangerous and you cannot be electrocuted!

What does an exercise ECG involve?

An exercise ECG records the electrical activity of your heart
when you are walking on a treadmill (or bicycle) exercise
machine (Figure 3.3); in other words, it imitates you walking in
the street or uphill, when the effect of any coronary narrowing is
most likely to show up. It is used to help your doctor when
unsure whether you have angina or, if you have angina, to decide
whether it is severe or not.

The test speeds up every 3 minutes and the uphill slope is
increased to give your heart a gradual stress. The doctor looks for

any changes on the ECG, whether you are getting chest pains or are unduly short of breath, and an eye is kept on your blood pressure. Whilst on the treadmill, tell the doctor or technician if you have any pain or discomfort, or if you feel light-headed or sweaty. When the machine is stopped, the heart rate is monitored for another 5 minutes or so to see what happens.

I have an appointment for an exercise ECG. How should I prepare for it?

Wear comfortable shoes and loose clothing. Do not eat a meal or have caffeine drinks for 2 hours beforehand. Bring along any medication you are taking, including your nitrate tablets (see section on *Treatment* below). If you have a cold or 'flu, tell your doctor so that he or she can postpone the test.

My last week's ECG was absolutely normal. However, because the doctor still thinks that I have angina, I have got to go for more tests. Why?

You probably had an ECG at rest (lying down) and, if this was normal, it does not rule out coronary artery disease. It can be falsely reassuring, so an exercise ECG is usually advised. If the ECG is abnormal at rest or on exercise, you may then need further tests to try and find out if coronary narrowing exists and how severe it is.

What makes the exercise test abnormal?

An exercise test may suggest that you have coronary artery disease if the ECG changes, if you get pain of a certain kind or out of breath, or if your blood pressure falls. As a rule the longer you can keep going, the better: 9 minutes is average and 12 minutes or more is good. The doctor will tell you the result of the test in the clinic and he or she may make recommendations for treatment or further tests. If you get pain or your ECG shows changes in less than 6 minutes, then this is a strong sign that you have narrowed arteries and need specialized treatment.

Angiogram

**I have been told to go to the hospital for an angiogram.
What is this and what does it involve?**

A coronary angiogram (pronounced *ann-gee-o-gram*) is also
known as cardiac catheterization. This is a technique for
establishing if there are any narrowings in your coronary arteries,
how severe they are and whether they represent an increased risk
of heart attack (see Figure 3.4). If narrowings are severe and in
dangerous places, the doctor will then know that surgery is the
best treatment for you. An angiogram can also give information
about the heart valves and the quality of the muscle pump (left
ventricle) and whether there is any damage.

The test involves small tubes (catheters) being passed through
your arteries. Special X-rays are then taken of the coronary
arteries and the heart muscle. When a dye is injected into the
tube, any narrowings will be shown and any danger discovered.
This test is straightforward but only done when there is a
probability of narrowing that could be corrected by an operation
or by the technique of *angioplasty* (see question later on
Percutaneous transluminal coronary angioplasty).

You will usually be in and out the same day. You will be given a
ward bed and have nothing to eat or drink for 4 hours before the
test as, just occasionally, the dye used to show up the arteries can
make people feel sick.

You may be given medicine to help you relax. You will be taken
to the catheter laboratory usually by a porter or a nurse. Some
hospitals use trolleys, others wheelchairs and, in many, you
simply walk down with the nurse. The laboratory nurses will
introduce themselves and you will meet the cardiologist who is
doing the angiogram. The 'cath lab' is full of sophisticated
equipment all designed to help diagnose your problem.

You will asked to lie on a table (usually it is rather hard!)
beneath an X-ray camera, which will make a noise when in use.
TV screens will show the procedure as it's happening, so that you
can watch what's going on (if you want to).

There are two ways of doing the angiogram – one from the arm and one from the leg. Most procedures are done from the leg, but different hospitals have different procedures, and some people may not be suitable for the leg procedure because of hardened leg arteries.

A local anaesthetic is applied to the top of your leg and you will feel a needle prick followed by a stinging numbing sensation. This is the only discomfort that you should feel. A fine tube is passed through the artery all the way to your heart. You will not feel this tube. Once the tube (the catheter) is safely in place, dye is injected into the arteries and the ventricle (pumping chamber) and pictures will be taken. You will hear the camera run several times as pictures are taken from different angles, and the camera will move over your chest to the left and right. Imagine your arteries to the heart are like a big tree and that you are walking around the bottom looking up at all the big and little branches; as you move around, any area of overlap becomes clear. So it is with the camera: it moves to unravel the branches so that nothing is missed. You may be asked to hold your breath from time to time and your arms may be put over your head if they are in the camera's way.

The whole procedure usually takes less than 30 minutes and often only 10–15 minutes.

Is there any difference between an angiogram from the arm or the leg?

The leg approach does not involve stitches but pressure is needed for 10 minutes or so to stop the bleeding (a tiny hole is made in the artery by a fine needle). To prevent re-bleeding, you will be advised bed rest for 4–6 hours. This technique is *percutaneous* which means 'through the skin' but no surgical cut is involved. Devices have been developed to 'plug' the hole in the artery and, if you are a suitable candidate, the artery will be closed and you will not need pressure on the groin. You will rest in bed for about an hour and then get up and about, going home sooner.

The arm approach is usually percutaneous at the wrist (radial artery) and does not need bed or chair rest for more than an hour.

The arm approach at the elbow can be percutaneous but often

A blockage here
affects a large area
of the heart

A blockage here involves only
a small area of the heart

Figure 3.4 The relative risks of coronary artery blockage.

needs a cut and then stitches (the jargon we use is cut-down). Again mobilisation is rapid. The wrist and leg techniques are the most common.

I have been on warfarin tablets for some time now, to prevent blood clots. Do I need to stop or reduce my warfarin before the angiogram?

Warfarin is a medication used to prevent blood clots from forming. It is not always necessary to stop or reduce warfarin with the arm approaches, but it is essential with the leg approach to prevent severe bruising. We usually advise four days of no therapy before an angiogram. Always remind the doctor that you are taking warfarin so your clotting can be checked before the procedure.

I'm taking aspirin every day – do I need to stop this for the angiogram?

No, this is not necessary. The mild blood-thinning action of aspirin helps prevent clotting in the artery narrowings but it does not usually significantly increase the tendency to bruising or bleeding. This answer applies if you are taking clopidogrel as an alternative to aspirin.

Is the angiogram at all painful?

The only discomfort should be the injection of local anaesthetic. When the dye is injected into your muscle pump, you may feel hot and flushed with a strange warm feeling in your bottom. This passes quickly. Sometimes when the catheter is in the pumping chamber, your heart may appear to miss a beat or flutter for a few seconds. Don't be afraid; this is all routine.

After the procedure pressure will be applied to your groin to stop the bleeding (about 15 minutes) and you will be asked to rest in bed for 4–6 hours while the small hole in your artery closes. If your arm has been used, a pressure bandage will be applied to your wrist.

Is the angiogram procedure dangerous?

All tests have a slight risk but in an experienced centre the complication rate is about 1 in a 1000. Remember that this figure includes emergency and sick people as well as people undergoing routine tests. The test is never done without a good reason and the risks are very low.

What happens after I have had my angiogram?

Your ward nurse will collect you from the 'cath' department and take you back to your bed on the ward. If you have had an angiogram by the leg approach, until you are safely back in bed, you may be asked to press on the leg used and to keep it as straight as possible. This is to prevent further bleeding from the site. This rarely happens but, if it does, don't panic; press as the nurse or doctor did and call for help.

Your nurse will record your pulse and blood pressure at frequent intervals to check that all is well. The site of the catheter insertion will be checked and the pulses felt in your feet or arm. If you notice any blood, apply pressure as before and tell your nurse. If your arm or leg feels cold, also tell the nurse.

If the arm has been used, you will get up almost straight away but, if the leg is used or a 'plug' has not been inserted, you will be asked to remain in bed for 4–6 hours, still keeping that leg straight. When you wish to go to the toilet, the nurse will bring the urinal or bedpan. If you have had a leg angiogram, you can usually get out of bed after 4–6 hours (1–2 hours if a plug has been inserted). Check when it is safe to get up. Don't get up without checking first.

How long after my angiogram will I get my results?

When your films have been developed and studied, the doctors will come to discuss the results of your angiogram with you, usually the same day. Some hospitals have a weekly conference so there may be a delay. Any further treatment that you may need, either medical or surgical, will then be discussed with you, either before you go home or in the outpatient clinic after the conference.

If the coronary arteries are hardened, the doctor will be able to show you your results by means of a diagram.

What happens after I have been discharged from hospital, following the angiogram?

Problems are rare. Sometimes the leg is bruised but this slowly fades over 2–3 weeks. Occasionally a hard lump, like a gland, is felt in the groin: this is just a bruise again. Don't worry – if it is tender, take pain killers.

Have a quiet evening when you get home, but you can be up

and about the next day. Any sticking plaster is best removed in the bath the following morning. If you have had a leg angiogram, you should avoid strenuous exercise for 48 hours. If you have had an arm cut-down angiogram, you need to make arrangements for stitch removal if the non-dissolvable sort have been used – your family doctor will do this at about seven days. If pain continues or the scar looks red and swollen, go to your doctor. It is unusual, but infection can occur and antibiotics will then be needed.

If you are taking warfarin, you should start your tablets again the same day, although it is a good plan to confirm this with the hospital doctor before leaving. Those who work can get back to work usually in a couple of days; driving is possible also the next day.

I always thought that angina was a man's problem. Do women get angina?

Coronary disease is the most important cause of death and disability in women. It is six times more likely to cause premature death in women than breast cancer. Angina is just as much a woman's problem as a man's (see section on **Women and coronary artery disease** in Chapter 2).

I have had my angiogram and my arteries are clear, but I still have angina. My doctor says that I have Syndrome X – what does this mean?

This is a condition which is more common in women. There is no extra risk of a heart attack or dropping dead, but nearly two-thirds of people with chest pain and normal arteries who suffer from angina are significantly limited by it. It is very difficult to treat. Drugs that relax the arteries to try and improve the blood flow (nitrates, calcium antagonists, nicorandil) may help. It is important to rule out other problems that may mimic angina, in particular a hiatus hernia or excess stomach acid.

People who suffer from Syndrome X can help themselves by:

- not smoking

- exercising as much as possible, and

- reducing weight if they are overweight.

It is a very frustrating condition to treat and we do not have all the answers – some people are helped, some are not. It is important, however, not to give up trying to help. It is a real condition and not 'in the mind'.

Treatment

What is there, apart from medication, to treat angina?

Relief measures other than medication include angioplasty and surgery. First, there are some general self-help measures. These have been discussed before but to summarize:

- Stop smoking.

- Lose weight.

- Cut down on alcohol.

- Take exercise.

- Take life easier by reducing stress.

The use of aspirin as a preventative drug has been discussed a lot in the media recently. What does aspirin do?

Aspirin helps stop blood clotting. It reduces by 25% the risk of a heart attack and helps prevent strokes in people with angina or who have had a heart attack. You only need 75 mg a day and should not take more, unless specified by your doctor; 75 mg is a quarter of an adult 300 mg tablet. It occasionally upsets the stomach and a small number of people with asthma or bronchitis may be sensitive to it (it worsens the wheezing). Overall it is cheap, safe and very effective. Special types of coated aspirin are

Table 3.2 Drugs for angina

Generic name	Trade name
Nitrates	
Isosorbide mononitrate	Elantan, Imdur, Ismo, Monit, Mono-Cedocard
Glyceryl trintrate (tablets or spray)	
Beta blockers	
Atenolol	Tenormin, Totamol
Acebutolol	Sectral
Bisoprolol	Monocor, Emcor
Metoprolol	Betaloc, Lopresor
Nadolol	Corgard
Oxprenolol	Trasicor
Pindolol	Visken
Propranolol	Inderal, Beta-Prograne
Timolol	Betim, Blocadren
Calcium antagonists	
Amlodipine	Istin
Diltiazem	Adizem, Dilzem, Tildiem
Felodipine	Plendil
Nicardipine	Cardene
Nifedipine	Adalat, Adalat LA, Cardilate MR, Coracten XL
Nisoldipine	Syscor MR
Verapamil	Cordilox, Securon, Univer
Potassium channel activators	
Nicorandil	Ikorel

available for those who get indigestion but they are not always helpful. Taking a compound like Alkaseltzer is another way of taking aspirin and reducing the chances of a stomach upset; it contains 324 mg aspirin, so you will need to take only a quarter.

I get indigestion on aspirin – is there an alternative?

Clopidogrel (Plavix) 75 mg daily thins the blood to the same degree as aspirin and is used as an alternative. It is only available on prescription.

Medication

What relieves the pain of angina? Do I have to take medication?

Angina is relieved after 1–2 minutes by slowing down or stopping activity, or using a nitrate tablet or spray, usually GTN, short for glyceryl trinitrate. If you get pain on walking after a meal and stop to take an indigestion tablet, it will seem as if the tablet has helped. In fact it was the stopping that relieved the pain: this is often how angina and indigestion get confused.

Several drugs are available to stop angina occurring or to deal with an attack. We have already discussed cholesterol-lowering diets and tablets in Chapter 2 and it is essential that people with angina have a cholesterol test and know the result.

Anyone with angina should be prescribed and told how to use sublingual (under the tongue) nitrates and aspirin or clopidogrel. The other medications – oral nitrates, beta-blockers, calcium antagonists and potassium channel activators (discussed below) – are prescribed as necessary. See Table 3.2 for a list of currently available medications. Check the trade name against the generic name.

Nitrates

How do the nitrates work?

Nitrates open up the arteries by relaxing the muscle in the artery wall. They relax the coronary arteries to improve the blood flow; by relaxing the peripheral arteries (e. g. in the legs) and veins, they reduce the work the heart has to do. As the problem is one of too much demand and too little supply, nitrates attempt to rectify the situation by improving supply (by dilating the artery) and reducing demand (the heart pumps against less resistance as the arteries are relaxed).

My mother has been given sublingual nitrates but seems unclear what to do. As I am her carer, what do I need to know?

Sublingual nitrates are taken in tablet or spray form and are absorbed via the veins under the tongue. They are effective in 1–2 minutes and last 20–30 minutes. They relieve attacks and can be used when your mother fears an attack; for example, she can use them at the bottom of a hill before she starts to climb. Headache is the main side effect.

After collection from the chemist, tablets last only about 8 weeks and have to be stored correctly:

- Keep the tablets in the airtight bottle in which they have been dispensed.

- After use, close the bottle tightly.

- Do not put cottonwool, other tablets, or anything else in the bottle with these tablets.

- Store the tablets in a cool place. When your mother carries them with her, tell her not to put them too close to the heat of her body – she could keep them in a purse or handbag (other people can carry them in a briefcase).

- If she does not use the tablets within 8 weeks of opening the bottle, get a fresh supply and discard the old tablets. An active tablet produces a slight burning sensation when placed under the tongue. If this does not happen, you should get a fresh supply for her.

The spray lasts 2–3 years but is more expensive. It is useful when attacks are infrequent as it lasts longer in storage Tablets can be bought over the counter without prescription whereas the spray needs a doctor's prescription.

I have been given nitrate tablets to swallow. Are these different from the sublingual ones?

Yes, nitrates also come as tablets that are swallowed once or twice daily and can be taken on a regular basis to reduce your angina attacks and improve your ability to take exercise. The commonest are isosorbide mononitrate which are taken twice daily, or in slow release formulations (Imdur, Elantan, Monit SR) once daily. They must not be taken more often or the body gets used to them – known as tolerance – and they are then ineffective in relieving angina. Sublingual tablets are only taken when you have or fear an angina attack coming on.

There are also nitrate patches which are effective when placed on the skin like a plaster; they have to be taken off after 12 hours or your body again develops tolerance. Used 12 hours on and 12 hours off, they act as a back-up and can be helpful overnight if put on in the evening and taken off in the morning. They should not be used on their own because, with 12 hours off, no angina protection is provided for that period.

Since I have been taking nitrates for my angina, I seem to get headaches. Is this due to my medication and are there any other side effects?

Headache is certainly the most frequent side effect. Occasionally you may get palpitations (see Chapter 6) or flushing and sometimes the tablets under your tongue make your breath smell. Rarely, and particularly if the tablets are taken within a short while of drinking alcohol or when starving, you might get a dizzy attack, caused by a temporary lowering of blood pressure. If headaches are a problem, the nitrates will be stopped and other drugs substituted.

Beta-blockers

I have been prescribed beta-blockers for my angina. What are these?

These are very important medications. They are the only ones (besides aspirin, cholesterol-lowering tablets and ACE inhibitors) that have been medically proved to lengthen the life of many people with heart problems. Beta-blockers reduce the work that the heart has to do by slowing the heart rate and lowering the blood pressure. They also reduce the force with which the heart muscle contracts, so that it needs less energy. By slowing the heart rate, they allow more time for blood to flow to the heart past the narrowings, and they blunt the heart rate's response to exercise. If you were to run for a bus, your heart rate might rise to 130 beats per min (bpm); with a beta-blocker it might not get above 110 bpm, so you would be less likely to develop angina. A slower heart rate is therefore a feature of beta-blocker treatment and one of the main reasons that they are so effective in reducing the number of attacks that people experience, as well as allowing them to walk further. They also help people to live longer after a heart attack and may therefore help protect people with angina from serious complications.

Beta-blockers are swallowed, once or twice daily. The commonest in use are atenolol and bisoprolol but a large number exist. They should never be stopped suddenly because the heart can rebound the other way, and this can lead to severe bouts of chest pain or even a heart attack.

I have been taking beta-blockers regularly. Are there any side effects with this treatment?

Yes, beta-blockers can cause:

- wheezing (they should not be given to asthmatics);
- breathlessness and fatigue (general tiredness with feelings of being 'worn out' or 'washed out');
- cold hands and feet and heavy leg muscles (by slowing the circulation);
- muzzy head with poor concentration and vivid dreams;
- rarely, depression;
- occasional erection problems in men and reduced sex drive in women.

Do not stop taking your medication if you experience any of these effects. Tell your doctor and your tablets can be changed.

I have been very forgetful lately. Do you think this could be due to the beta-blockers I am taking? Are there any others I could take?

Yes. Some beta-blockers are soluble in water and do not cross into the brain (e. g. atenolol), so dreams and confusion or forgetfulness are less common. These are known as hydrophilic (dissolve in water) types. Others are soluble in fat (lipophilic) (e. g. propranolol) and can cross into the brain. Although you may have more side effects with propranolol, you may also find that you are less anxious.

I have noticed that I have a slight tremor. Can beta-blockers relieve tremor and shakiness?

Yes, beta-blockers can be very effective, particularly propranolol, if you have tremor. As a result they can also help people with Parkinson's disease. It is also claimed that they improve the performance of snooker players and golfers! This is likely where tremor is a major problem, of course, but the routine use of beta-blockers to improve performance is not approved of!

If my pulse drops below 50, should I stop taking my beta-blockers?

No. Beta-blockers act to slow the heart. The coronary arteries receive their oxygen and food between the beats, so the slower the rate, the more time the heart has to receive its food supply.

Your treatment will only be stopped if, owing to your slow heart rate, your symptoms of lethargy and fatigue become a problem. It is best to reduce the dose first. Do not stop any treatment without your doctor's advice. Beta-blockers should certainly not be stopped suddenly as this can cause a rebound chest pain and could be very dangerous.

When is the best time to take beta-blockers?

The once a day variety such as atenolol or bisoprolol are useful for people who have problems in remembering to take tablets (see question later in this section), and these are often best taken at night. This is a useful time to take them if they make you feel drowsy.

Is it a disaster if I forget to collect my prescription and run out of tablets?

You must try not to run out of your tablets as you may get rebound chest pain. Your chemist will give you some until you get your prescription renewed: it is dangerous to stop beta-blockers suddenly (see question above about stopping tablets suddenly).

My doctor prescribed beta-blockers some time ago and now has put me on nitrates as well. Is this safe?

Yes, the combination is very effective. For example, you may be given atenolol plus Imdur.

Calcium antagonists

What are calcium antagonists (calcium blockers)?

Calcium is an ion (an electrically charged particle) which increases the tone of muscles and strengthens the contraction of the muscle. The muscle in the wall of the artery depends on calcium for its tone, so if the movement of calcium into the muscle cell is 'antagonized' or 'blocked', the muscle will relax. As the muscle relaxes the artery becomes bigger, blood flow increases and the demands on the heart decrease.

Do calcium antagonists act in the same way as nitrates?

In a way, yes. They both increase the size of arteries but by different mechanisms. In combination they may have an additive effect, so you may be prescribed both.

Can I take calcium antagonists with beta-blockers?

Only some calcium antagonists. Verapamil must never be taken with a beta-blocker because of the danger of slowing the heart too dramatically. Diltiazem is used cautiously by some hospitals. Amlodipine, felodipine and nifedipine are quite safe and effective in combination with beta-blockers. Never mix your medications without first checking with your doctor or pharmacist.

I have not got on well with verapamil so my doctor plans to change my medication to nifedipine. Are there differences between the various types of calcium antagonists?

There are several calcium antagonists on the market and they have some differences which are important. Verapamil and diltiazem slow the heart rate as well as widening blood vessels, so they are a good alternative to beta-blockers, if beta-blockers are not suitable for you (e. g. if you have asthma) or they are giving you unacceptable side effects. Amlodipine, felodipine and nifedipine do not slow your heart rate and are often used in combination with beta-blockers.

Will I experience any side effects with calcium antagonists?

There are plenty of calcium antagonists on the market, so if you are prescribed one that does not suit you, tell your doctor so that your medication can be changed. Two common effects you are likely to experience are headaches and flushing because these medications open up the arteries.

Another common side effect is swollen ankles and this does

not respond to water tablets (diuretics) (see the section on **Treatment** in Chapter 5). Ankle swelling may improve as the dose is decreased but often the tablets have to be discontinued. Verapamil and diltiazem are less likely to lead to swollen ankles.

Constipation can be a problem if you are taking verapamil (and more so the older you get). High-fibre diets and lactulose can help but, if constipation becomes a serious problem, your doctor will change you onto another type of calcium antagonist.

Rarely, eye pain and gum problems occur. Calcium antagonists do not usually cause the tiredness that can be a problem with the beta-blockers. They may be less effective if you continue to smoke, whereas beta-blocker treatment is not affected by smoking. (Remember smoking causes heart attacks and can kill you.)

Why did my doctor prescribe beta-blockers for me rather than calcium antagonists?

Usually calcium antagonists are prescribed only if beta-blockers are not suitable or giving side effects. Some calcium antagonists can be combined with beta-blockers to give an additional benefit and all of them can be combined with nitrates (see question above about combining these medications).

I have found that beta-blockers have given me an unfortunate problem, in affecting my love life. My doctor says he will try me on calcium antagonists, but not straight away. Why not?

Your doctor will do this gradually. The beta-blocker must be wound down and the calcium antagonist wound up over a period of time. Calcium antagonists do not give you protection when beta-blockers are suddenly stopped.

Potassium channel activators

I seem to have been given all sorts of medication for my angina over time. My doctor has now said he wants me to try a new type called a potassium channel activator. I have never heard of this one! Will it do any good?

These are medications which work half like a nitrate and half like a calcium antagonist. There is only one available at the moment – nicorandil. It can be used on its own or in combination with the other three types of medication for angina (see Table 3.2). It does not cause swollen ankles, but headaches can be a problem. It is as good as the other medications but not any better, and it is very expensive in comparison. It tends to be used after the other options have been tried and in this way can be very helpful. So if you have tried all the other options, you might –with luck – find that this suits you.

Taking your medication

I am rather confused over the various medications available for angina. How many can I take at any one time?

Quite often, too many are taken at any one time! You will need aspirin and, usually, a cholesterol-lowering tablet (usually a statin) to reduce your chances of the coronary narrowings becoming worse. If one angina drug doesn't work, there is a tendency among doctors to add other medications rather than change the combination. If one drug partly works, it makes sense to increase its strength or add another in but, if it's not working, it makes no sense to continue it. There is no medical evidence that taking more than two medications for angina is better than one or two used properly. Many people could have their medication simplified, and it is possible that your doctor does not know exactly what you are taking, so always take all your tablets when you visit the surgery. If you are on many different tablets, discuss their strengths with your doctor and whether all of them are necessary. Do not make changes on your own. Many medications, taken twice or three times a day, are now in once-a-day formulations which makes life easier.

I am bad at remembering to take tablets. What should I do?

If you are on frequent doses (say three times a day), ask for a once-a-day alternative. For example, if you are on diltiazem 60 mg three times a day and isosorbide mononitrate 20 mg twice a day (five tablets), this could be changed to long-acting diltiazem 200 mg once a day and long-acting mononitrate once a day (i. e. two tablets altogether) with the same effect. Beta-blockers are often best taken at night. Any sedative side effects can then be slept off.

Try to establish a routine. Take your medication at the same time of day – with your morning cup of tea or after brushing your teeth. If you are on a lot of tablets, special pill boxes are available, such as the Dosette, that are split into time of day and days of the week (ask your pharmacist about these). Ask your partner or friends to remind you or stick reminders by the phone or on the fridge (use one of those reminder magnets).

Remember not to run out (see a previous question on this). If you have a question about your medication write it down – most people forget when they go to the doctor. It's a good idea to ask what each tablet is for and when you should take it. And remember to take all your tablets with you to the surgery – the doctor may not know what you are taking.

If you miss a dose of beta-blockers, take an extra tablet to catch up – others do not need boosting so just get back on schedule.

I have been told that cold remedies react with angina tablets. What can I do if I need them?

Some of these medications react, some don't. Show your heart tablets to the pharmacist and ask for advice about what you can or cannot take.

Am I allowed to drink alcohol with the medication?

Yes. However, alcohol does widen blood vessels, so the effects
may add up with those of nitrates and calcium antagonists to give
you more chance of a headache.

Are there any special dietary precautions that I should take while I am on angina medications?

The only precaution is to avoid grapefruit juice as it reacts with
some medications in the liver – especially calcium antagonists.

Are there any new medications for angina in the pipeline?

There are always new ones coming along. Most are variations on
what we have already. We always need to see whether they are
better than what we have or whether they can be added in to
improve what we have. Always beware of exaggerated claims and
look carefully at any statistics that are given. Above all,
remember that only beta-blockers have been proved to lengthen
your life.

I have heard that a drug call trimetazidine is available – what is this?

Trimetazidine is an interesting drug and acts to improve oxygen
supply by affecting how the cells of the heart work. It does not
affect heart rate or blood pressure. It is not available (unless
specially requested) in the UK but it is widely available
elsewhere. It is an effective drug with minimal indigestion side
effects and can be combined with all the other drugs available. It
is the first of a class of drugs known as 'metabolic agents'
because of its action improving how the cells function.
Ranolozine is another drug being developed.

Surgery

Angioplasty

I have been told that I need an angioplasty. What is this?

Percutaneous transluminal coronary angioplasty (PTCA) is a method of using a balloon to squash or push the arterial narrowings out of the way. (The medical word for these narrowings is *stenosis*, pronounced *sten-oh-siss.*) PTCA is often shortened to 'angioplasty'.

It is performed in the catheter laboratory usually by the same team who does the angiograms (see the section on ***Angiograms*** above) so you may meet some familiar faces. The doctor doing the operation will be the cardiologist, with whom you may already have had a consultation.

After a local anaesthetic, a thin tube (the catheter) is inserted into your artery at the top of your leg, or occasionally in an artery in your arm either at the elbow (brachial artery) or, more frequently, the wrist (radial artery). The catheter is guided under X-ray control to the heart, up the main artery known as the aorta (see Chapter 1). You cannot feel the tube moving. It is then directed into the coronary artery that contains the narrowing. This catheter is called the guide catheter. A very fine wire (the guidewire) is now passed up through this catheter and into the coronary artery where it is steered past the narrowing. This may be a bit fiddly. Once it is across the narrowing, the balloon catheter is passed along the wire (like a monorail) and, following the wire, it slides across the narrowing. The balloon is blown up (inflated) once it is in position. This may cause some chest pain – let the doctor know if you have any pain at all.

The pressure in the balloon is increased and the narrowed part is pushed back into the wall of the artery where it has come from. The result is checked after the balloon has been deflated and removed back into the guide catheter. At this point the wire is still in place so that the balloon can be used again, or exchanged for a bigger balloon, if the result needs to be improved.

Once the doctor is satisfied with the result, the balloon and wire are removed; and you will be given a dye injection which checks how well the operation has gone; the guide catheter is then removed (Figure 3.5).

A small insertion sheath is left in the groin for about four hours, because the effects of blood thinning medication (heparin), used to prevent clotting on the wire or balloon, need to wear off. The sheath is removed on the ward and the groin pressed firmly for 20 minutes or so. If the radial artery (at the wrist) is used, it is firmly bandaged. Occasionally, the leg artery is plugged so that you can get up and about more quickly.

I am rather worried about the PTCA procedure. Will I be given any relaxing medicine beforehand?

This depends on you and how you are feeling. If you are anxious, then an injection of diazepam (Diazemuls or Valium) helps you to relax.

Will I feel any pain when I undergo PTCA?

The local anaesthetic stings rather like when you have an angiogram. When the balloon is inflated, it blocks the artery temporarily (usually for a minute or so), so you may get some chest pain. Let the doctor know if you are feeling any pain.

How long does the PTCA procedure last? Will I need to be in hospital for long?

Some procedures are quick (5–10 minutes), others take up to 1 hour. It depends on the number of narrowings in your particular case, whether they can be reached easily and whether you need a stent (see questions below on stents) or not.

Usually you will be in hospital for one night. This is the big advantage over bypass surgery (see the question later on bypass surgery) – you don't have to spend long in hospital and you recuperate rapidly.

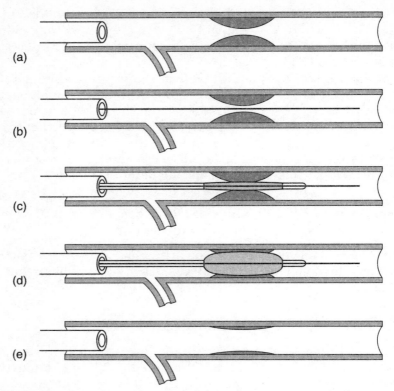

Figure 3.5 Figure 3.5 The technique of angioplasty. (**a**) Guide catheter in left coronary artery. (**b**) Guidewire advanced through narrowing. (**c**) Balloon positioned with markers. (**d**) Balloon inflated. (**e**) Catheter, with guidewire and balloon, removed leaving expanded artery.

How long will the effects of PTCA last?

In seven cases out of 10, PTCA gives a complete cure. However, for reasons we don't understand fully, 30% of the narrowings come back in about 4–6 months. You will only know that the operation has not been entirely successful because your angina will return.

If my angina returns, can the PTCA be repeated?

Yes – up to five or six times, and each time it is performed, you have a seven out of 10 chance of it remaining successful.

If you have no angina after 6 months, the effects will last for years, so the first 6 months constitute an important hurdle to overcome.

Can the cardiologist perform PTCA on more than one narrowing at a time?

Yes, as many as are necessary (but see the question below on unsuitable narrowings). Sometimes the procedure may be staged so that you come back for other narrowings to be done on a separate occasion. This decision depends on the importance of each narrowing and whether the procedure was an emergency or not – in an emergency only the most dangerous narrowing is done (the culprit), and the rest are completed when matters have settled down.

I am worried that things may go wrong when I have my PTCA. Is this likely?

Things are very unlikely to go wrong but, if they do not work out, there are other ways to sort out the problem. Complications are not common but they do occur. Sometimes the artery tears and closes completely. We can correct this by inserting a stent or moving on to bypass surgery (see below). However, angioplasty is successful over 95% of the time. You will be asked to sign a form giving your consent to having a stent inserted or bypass surgery, just in case the PTCA is not successful.

I have been told that I am not suitable for PTCA. Why is this?

Some people have complicated narrowings and complete blockages which unfortunately are not suitable for PTCA. If you suffer from angina and many arteries are affected, a coronary bypass (see the question later on bypass surgery) may be the best option for you.

When my husband went into hospital for a PTCA, he had to sign a form saying he consented to having a stent inserted if it was found necessary during the operation. What is a stent and how does it work?

A stent is a metal mesh cage rather like a small spring. It is made of thin flexible metal wire and is fixed to a balloon with the balloon deflated. The original angioplasty balloon is removed – the wire is still in the artery so we have access to the narrowing – and the balloon with the stent on it is passed along the wire to the narrowing. The balloon inside the stent is inflated and the stent expands to the size of the balloon. It embeds itself into the artery wall and holds the artery open mechanically. The balloon is deflated and removed but the stent is permanently left behind (Figure 3.6). More than one stent may be used and the stent sizes vary according to the size of the arteries.

When will the cardiologist decide to insert a stent?

There are various reasons why the cardiologist decides to use a stent. The commonest are:

- if the angioplasty is not successful or the artery closes off;
- out of choice;
- if the narrowing comes back 4–6 months after angioplasty;
- if the artery is large and the narrowing short, as the recurrence rate is reduced to 10–15%.
- if the narrowing is within a vein used for coronary bypass.

Stents are now used in over 85% of cases because of the better long-term results with only 15% getting a narrowing within the stent after 6 months (this figure rises to 30% with the balloon). If possible, they are placed directly without using a balloon beforehand as this reduces the risk of a complication.

Figure 3.6 The technique of stent insertion. (**a**) The stent (like a metal cage) on balloon catheter is positioned at the problem site. (**b**) The balloon catheter is then inflated. (**c**) The stent is fully expanded and (**d**) left in place after the balloon has been deflated. (**e**) The stent remains expanded inside the artery.

Drug-eluting stents have been developed and are claimed to have a better than 95% long-term success. These have a drug coated on the metal stent, which acts to stop any further narrowing occurring. They are much more expensive than ordinary stents but obviously reduce the chances of a repeat procedure. They may be particularly important in higher risk cases for a recurrence – those who have had a recurrence already, people with diabetes, and when the artery being stented is small.

I need an MRI scan. Do I tell the radiologist about my stents?

Yes. Routine MRI scanning is safe in all patients who have had a stent in place for 6 weeks. Stainless steel stents may displace in the first 6 weeks, but other makes remain secure. The chances of a stainless steel stent moving are, however, minimal so that MRI in an emergency should go ahead. Non-urgent cases should play safe and wait 6 weeks.

I was not offered a stent as a choice. Why was this?

This is most likely because angioplasty alone gave an excellent result. Stents are not as successful in smaller arteries, so this may have been the reason. Sometimes the arteries are too tortuous to allow a stent to pass through.

I am on tablets only at the moment for my angina. Is angioplasty or stenting better than medications?

Angioplasty or stenting can relieve any pain that medications have failed to control. They do not, however, provide any benefits compared to medication for preventing heart attacks. They are used only if conventional medical treatment does not give you relief from pain and a good quality of life. Angioplasty is a safe and effective procedure, but any operation has a slight risk, which you should avoid if possible.

I have been told that I need an angioplasty. I would prefer not to have an operation. Am I being overcautious?

Probably not. Because a narrowing looks suitable for a balloon, that doesn't mean that it is the best treatment. Angina from a narrowing in a branch vessel that is not a danger to life will usually settle with drug treatment, and the angioplasty option can be saved for later. As angioplasty in research studies has not been shown to improve (or shorten) life expectancy, it must be used selectively and it is then a very effective procedure. Using any procedure in every circumstance invites complications and devalues what is a useful form of therapy.

I am worried about having angioplasty done. Is there any chance that I will not get through the operation?

You have a greater than 99% chance of survival. These statistics include emergency operations and very sick people – routine cases like you have a lower risk.

When will the doctor decide that I should have an angioplasty?

If you have angina and your tablets are not controlling it, the doctor will probably refer you for an angioplasty, if the narrowings are suitable. You will have an 80–90% chance of being relieved of your angina as a result.

I have just undergone an angioplasty with a stent and now been given some medication called clopidogrel. What is this drug for?

This is a powerful aspirin-like drug that prevents clotting on stents until they fully bed in. It is usually commenced about 6 hours before the procedure with a loading dose of 300 mg. You will take it for 2–4 weeks. Some doctors use it with aspirin also. Clopidogrel 75 mg daily is also used as an alternative in those unable to tolerate aspirin. Clopidogrel is also used in patients with unstable angina (see earlier section on *Symptoms*) as it reduces the complication rate. Skin rashes are the commonest side effect.

Drug-eluting stents can also clot and need the same treatment.

Now that I have had an angioplasty. which has cured me of my angina pain, can I throw away all those tablets?

No, not all! You will need to continue with aspirin, cholesterol-lowering tablets and blood pressure tablets, if necessary. Any tablets that you take for angina might be reduced or stopped. Ask your doctor first – do not stop any medication without advice.

My wife has just come out of hospital where she underwent an angioplasty. She wasn't allowed to drive herself home. Why?

A week off is recommended. If you are recovering satisfactorily, you can then start driving again. The DVLA need not be notified but car insurance companies must be informed. For Group II driving, see the question below.

I hold a Group II licence and drive a lorry for a living. Will I lose my job and livelihood after angioplasty?

Driving is not recommended anyway if you have angina, even if your symptoms are controlled on medical treatment. This is a safety rule to protect the general public in case you should lose control of the vehicle during an attack. If you have heart failure (see Chapter 4), the DVLA can refuse you a licence. After a heart attack, bypass or angioplasty, you should stop professional driving for 6 weeks and you will only be allowed to resume if you have no symptoms and are able to complete an exercise test to the required standard.

How many people who have undergone angioplasties or stent insertion will have to then have an urgent bypass operation?

Only about 1 in 100.

My doctor mentioned a PCI – what is this?

PCI stands for *percutaneous coronary intervention* and this term covers both balloons and stents.

Bypass surgery

I have had medication and lots of tests for angina. I am now being offered bypass surgery. Why do I need this?

Operations for coronary artery disease are usually designed to improve the blood supply to the heart. A decision by the consultant as to whether to advise an operation for you is based on your case history and on several special tests, including an electrocardiogram, an exercise test and an angiogram (see the section on *Angiogram* earlier in this chapter). This last test is the most crucial one for bypass operations as it demonstrates the exact position and extent of the narrowings. An operation may be advised on the basis of the severity of the symptoms or the extent of the disease or both – the operation may be performed to make you feel better, to prevent a heart attack or to correct life-shortening disease, thus giving you a longer and more active life.

Can you tell me what the bypass operation is all about?

The most common operation for angina is a coronary artery bypass. The full name is *coronary artery bypass graft* or CABG – often referred to as 'cabbage'.

A portion of vein is carefully removed from the leg and attached to the affected coronary artery beyond the narrowing. The other end of the vein is attached to the aorta, the main artery leading from the heart (see Chapter 1). In other words, the narrowing or obstruction is bypassed, just as a bypass can avoid bottlenecks in towns. Several of these vein grafts may be placed, often one to each of the three major coronary artery branches. Frequently the graft is made with the left and right mammary artery from inside the chest (Figure 3.7). The radial artery is more frequently used now and taken from your lower arm between the wrist and elbow. Artery bypasses are believed to be stronger and longer lasting than vein bypasses. In each case your body can put up with the loss of the vein or artery used for the bypass.

In order to do these operations, the surgeon requires your heart to stop beating; so the heart and lungs are rested while the

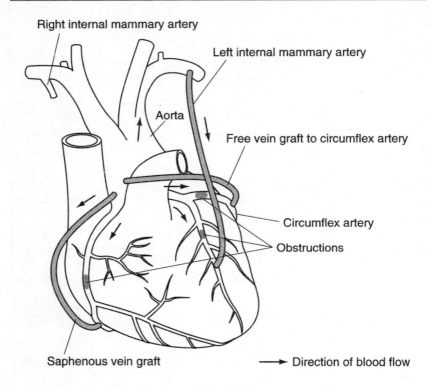

Figure 3.7 Diagram of coronary artery bypass surgery. Veins are used from the aorta to beyond the blockage and the mammary arteries taken directly from inside the chest.

body is kept going by a heart–lung bypass machine. The operation is carried out through an incision down the front of the chest.

I read that some people can have a bypass without the need for a heart-lung machine – is this keyhole surgery?

Not really keyhole, but in selected cases the bypass can be done with the heart still beating. This is known as 'off-pump'. In appropriate cases the results are good and there may be fewer complications. The surgeon will decide as to who is suitable, based on the angiogram and medical history.

I am rather confused about the differences between the cardiologist and the surgeon – aren't they same?

No. The cardiologist is a medical doctor who makes the diagnosis, investigates and treats you, and decides what is best to be done. The surgeon is the 'plumber' who puts in the bypasses and heart valves. When the job is done, the surgeon usually hands you back to the cardiologist to keep an eye on you. The cardiologist and surgeon work closely as a team to advise on and time the best treatment for you.

My doctor says that my heart has done its own bypass – what does he mean?

The coronary arteries link up through very small branches – they don't come to a full stop. This means that the left coronary artery can supply the right via the links, and vice versa. If these branches enlarge, they may fill a blocked artery backwards. This means, for example, that a blocked right coronary artery may get its blood supply from the left system. The enlarging arteries are known as *collaterals*. Collaterals develop over time and can be encouraged by regular exercise. If you 'develop collaterals'. so that a blocked artery gets its blood supply from another artery, it is then as if you have done your own bypass because, in effect, the blockage has been bypassed by your own arteries (Figure 3.8).

What do you use for a bypass operation if there are no suitable veins?

You have two arteries in the chest that can be used, two spare ones in the arms and also in the abdomen. The surgeon will find a way around the problem.

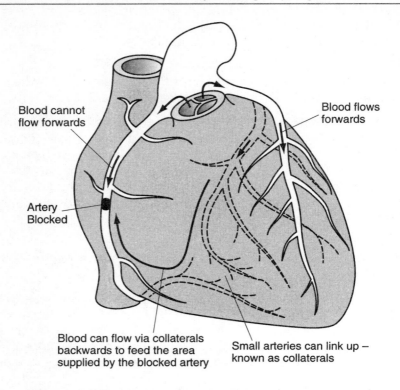

Blood cannot
flow forwards

Blood flows
forwards

Artery
Blocked

Blood can flow via collaterals
backwards to feed the area
supplied by the blocked artery

Small arteries can link up –
known as collaterals

Figure 3.8 Developing collaterals – doing your own bypass.

My doctor has recommended a bypass operation, but after all I've read about it, I don't think I want to have it done. Am I being used as a guineapig?

The risks of severe coronary artery disease are higher if you do nothing. It is always important to discuss your own risks so that you and your family will know where you stand. Risks will vary with age, how strong your heart muscle is and the extent of the coronary disease. On average 98 patients in 100 pull through and two therefore do not. So you have a 98% rate of success but, if you are one of the other 2%, you have a 100% chance of dying. The odds are heavily on your side but it is important to understand what the statistics mean – if, for example, I told you that, because the operation is difficult, you had a 98% chance of living, you would feel differently to hearing that you had a one in 50 chance of dying, even though the figures mean exactly the same!

How long will a bypass graft last?

It used to be said that bypass surgery lasted 10 years, but these figures are out of date. The mammary artery bypass has a better than 90% chance of working for longer than 15 years after surgery. The veins can still harden and narrow but, with the use of aspirin and cholesterol-lowering medication, the length of time these bypasses lasts is improving all the time. The success depends on dealing with those factors that you have some control over, in particular high cholesterol levels, smoking and high blood pressure.

What happens before the bypass operation?

The surgeon who is going to perform the operation will examine you and explain what is planned. It is a great help for you to have your teeth checked by your own dentist well beforehand so that last minute treatment can be avoided. This is to make sure there is no hidden infection that might affect the operation. Blood samples will be taken for tests; an electrocardiogram and a chest X-ray will also be taken. You will be visited by the physiotherapist and intensive care unit nursing staff to explain details of treatment to you. Before the operation, the anaesthetist will check on your lungs and ask about any allergies. The anaesthetist is a very important member of the team – your breathing will be controlled whilst the operation is being carried out.

Your chest and legs will be carefully shaved and you will be given a special antiseptic soap to clean the skin in several baths or showers. You will not have any food or drink for 4 hours before the anaesthetic is due. About 1 hour before the operation an injection will be given which will make you drowsy. The next thing you will know is waking up in the intensive care unit with the operation completed. The operation will take about 2–4 hours.

Why is the intensive care unit different to a normal ward?

The intensive care unit (ICU) is a halfway house between the operating theatre and the ward. You can be carefully observed there until you are again fit to be left to your own devices. Immediately after the operation you will still be fully anaesthetized and on a breathing machine. On awakening several hours later you will have a tube in your mouth attached to the breathing machine, so that for a little while you will not be able to speak properly. This can be frightening at first and frustrating. However, as soon as you are fully awake, the tube is removed. As you are likely to be very thirsty at this time, you may take sips of water. The ICU is busy and noisy with lots of sophisticated machines. They are all there to help you and make sure the operation is a success. You may find it hard to rest. As soon as the nursing staff consider that it is safe to do so, you will be transferred to the main ward. You may feel that you have lost a day or are 'jet-lagged' and it is easy to be confused, but matters soon right themselves and you will soon feel yourself again.

One of the first visitors to the ICU is the physiotherapist. During the operation there is a tendency for your bronchial tubes to collect sputum and become blocked, causing small areas of collapse in the lungs. These then have to be fully expanded again by deep breathing and coughing with the encouragement and assistance of the physiotherapist. Naturally, after such an operation, your chest will be sore and you may be somewhat anxious about exerting yourself. However, with proper pain-killing injections and tablets, and knowing that there is no danger of 'bursting' stitches, you will soon overcome this fear. Giving up smoking as long as possible before the operation will greatly help in this respect.

What happens on the normal ward when I get transferred?

As far as operations go, bypass surgery is not one of the most painful, but many people often complain of feeling a bit low in spirits for a few days afterwards. This is only temporary and may be accompanied by other symptoms such as fatigue, poor concentration, slight blurring of vision, loss of taste, a disturbance of sleep pattern with drowsiness during the day, and restlessness and sweating at night. All these symptoms very rapidly pass off and are no cause for alarm. If it hurts to cough, clutch a small pillow to your chest (or better still a teddy bear – a present for your recovery!).

If you become constipated, mention it to the Ward Sister who will provide a mild laxative.

After one or two days, you will be encouraged to get out of bed and walk about. People vary greatly in their speed of recovery and getting up and about. There are no set rules – so if someone else appears to be doing better than you, it does not mean that anything is wrong. There is no competition involved! The nurses and physiotherapists will encourage you to get on your feet as fast as you can manage it without exhaustion.

You will usually be given support stockings for your legs, to prevent swelling and to keep your circulation moving. It is important that, when you are resting, you keep your legs raised on a stool or in bed, to avoid swelling during the first few days.

After about six to seven days, any stitches will be removed from your chest and leg. You can have a bath if you want one. Leg wounds take longer than most to heal, and there may be a discharge of clear fluid, especially if your leg is not kept raised. This is not serious but should be pointed out to your doctor. It may feel a little numb just above the ankle on the inside of your leg.

Is it normal to get chest pains after the operation?

Muscular pains are common and can affect the chest, neck and back. They usually wear off over 2–3 weeks but can remind you of the operation for 2–3 months. Occasionally, bone and joint pain is a significant problem and anti-inflammatory tablets are prescribed. Most pains settle with simple painkillers, such as paracetamol or the stronger co-proxamol.

Can I lie on my side after a bypass operation?

You can lie in any position that you find comfortable.

Can the wound from a bypass operation fall apart?

No – your breastbone is wired together and you cannot undo the stitches or damage the operation. Very rarely the breastbone does not heal quickly and a click will be heard.

I am told that bypass surgery will make a large scar. Can't it be done by keyhole surgery?

Keyhole surgery is a media word – it does not happen in real life. In a few carefully selected cases, a bypass operation can be done without the need to open the breastbone or stop the heart. A cut is made to the side of the breastbone through three or four ribs and, whilst the heart is still beating, the surgeon constructs the bypass. Recovery is quicker than after a full bypass operation. It is a new procedure that is very appealing to the public, but applicable *only to a small number of people*, and it needs more testing to prove its effectiveness. If you are offered this option, ask about your particular surgeon's results and whether you will be entered in a research study to judge the success. Some surgeons are now opening only the lower end of the breastbone, which means that women can wear lower-cut garments, if they wish, without the scar showing.

I had a bypass some weeks ago. My scar is still tender. Why is this?

At the end of the operation, wires are used to pull the breastbone together and hold it firm for healing – these are not usually removed. It sounds as though you are one of the small number of people who feel the ends of these wire stitches. This may settle down or only be an occasional problem; however, occasionally they can give trouble. The problem can usually be pinpointed by pressing with a finger. If this problem occurs, the wires can be removed under anaesthesia by your surgeon, because once the breastbone has healed the wires are no longer necessary.

My chest scar is pink and overgrown, following my bypass operation. Can it be improved?

Occasionally, the operation scar may become pink and enlarges like a ridge. This is known as a *keloid*. It can be tender, itchy and unsightly. If it is a problem, steroid creams can be tried in order to relieve the discomfort. If it is intolerable, the scar can be cut out and then deep X-ray treatment given to stop the skin cells enlarging again.

I am due out of hospital in a few days after a successful bypass operation. What problems might I have?

Most people go straight home providing there is someone there to help. If you live alone, it is best to spend the first 2 weeks with relatives or friends but, if this is not possible, your doctor should arrange for your convalescence in a convalescent home, preferably before the operation. You will be given a supply of painkillers, a letter for your family doctor and advice on aspirin, diet and cholesterol medication. If you suffered from high blood pressure beforehand, this usually returns after the operation and will need careful checking. Almost certainly your blood pressure medications will need restarting.

When you return home, you may feel tired for a week or two. Although you are not exerting yourself, your body is doing a lot of repair work during this time.

How will I know that my bypass operation has been successful?

Your angina will be much less or non-existent. You will be less short of breath and have much more energy. You may say to yourself, 'I didn't realize how tired I had been', as you discover a new lease of life. A bypass should be a new start for you and your heart.

What exercise can I do on leaving hospital after my bypass operation?

Regarding exercise, you can do what you like within the bounds of commonsense! Unless carried to extremes, exercise will not hurt you. Any excess exercise will simply make you feel exhausted, and you can use this as a sign by which to pace yourself as you regain your fitness. In fact regular exercise is an important factor in rehabilitation (see Chapter 10).

There is no reason to avoid normal sexual activities (see Chapter 8). The main problem may be pain from the muscles in the chest. If there are any problems do not avoid the subject, ask for help from your own doctor. Hairs on men's chests are prickly when they regrow and their partners may find this uncomfortable. A small soft pillow placed over the chest between partners can help.

I have a small garden at home. I'm due for a bypass operation next month. When will I be able to start gardening again?

Gardening is a good rewarding exercise. Pace yourself doing the light work at first (weeding, dead-heading). Kneel down rather than bend over, to avoid muscular chest pain. Dig light soil but avoid the heavier clay soil until you are fully recovered. Cutting the grass should be possible after 3–4 weeks if the mower is light (such as a hover-type). Avoid heavy work (lifting bags of fertilizer) or pushing a heavy roller mower until 6–8 weeks, when you should be back to normal.

I have been told that I should go on a cardiac rehabilitation programme. What does this involve and do I really need it, now that I feel so much better?

These programmes are strongly recommended as they give you structured advice on exercise and help you get out and about to meet others; these gatherings are a great boost to your confidence. In fact, you should positively demand to go on one! If one is not offered to you, make enquiries from the hospital where you had the operation or, if this a long distance away, ask your doctor or local cardiac unit. Rehabilitation programmes have been proved to help you get back to a normal life quicker, and there is now evidence that, if you follow all the advice, you will prevent problems in the future. You discover that you are not alone and you will find help is plentiful and advice freely given.

Are rehabilitation programmes just about exercise?

No – they offer lots of general advice. They assess whether you are anxious or depressed, advise on stress and how to relax, and you can raise any concerns you might have for example about resuming sexual activity, diet or which medication you need to take.

Now that I am back home after my bypass operation, how soon can I start driving again?

You should be able to drive your car 4 weeks after the operation. Check first with your doctor. The DVLA does not need to be notified but your car insurance company does. If you drive a heavy goods vehicle, you will have to pass an exercise test 6 weeks after the operation (see section on Angioplasty).

I would like to have a holiday now that I have had my bypass – would this be a good idea?

Yes indeed. A period of relaxation in a warm climate helps recovery. Airlines prefer you to wait 6 weeks before travelling and this is a good time in your recovery as it helps you get back to full strength. If an emergency arises and you need to travel by plane before the 6 weeks, there is usually no problem, but you may need a doctor's letter saying that it is all right to travel. Some travel insurance companies also require a letter. At the airport, the wires in your chest do not usually set off the alarms, but as the equipment's sensitivity varies from airport to airport, you may rarely set the alarm off. Stents do not usually sound the alarms either, but pacemakers do (see Chapter 6). After an angioplasty or stent placement, you may travel sooner – even within a week, although the doctor usually advises waiting 7–14 days.

How soon can I go back to work after a bypass operation?

If you were able to work before the operation, you should be back at work 2–3 months later. If your job involved hard physical labour or long working hours, ideally you should try to find a less strenuous job However, hard physical work is safe if you become strong and fit again – ask the rehabilitation team to advise on strength-building exercises. If you are aged over 60 years of age, you should think about the possibility of early retirement if financially possible.

I feel very tired with angina and I am looking forward to having my bypass operation. Will I really feel better after surgery?

You should feel fitter and stronger with much less or no angina. Many people feel much less fatigued.

I didn't really see the purpose of bypass surgery, but am prepared to undergo it if I can guarantee avoiding this terrible pain. I couldn't bear the thought of the operation not working. How can I stop my angina returning later?

Follow the guidelines on weight, exercise and cholesterol in Chapter 2.

- Do not smoke.

- Make sure your blood pressure is normal and your cholesterol low. Your target LDL cholesterol should be below 3.0 and below 2.6 if possible. Once you have achieved this, keep it down. The target is lower for those who have undergone bypass surgery in order to protect the veins that have been used from narrowing and hardening.

- Take charge of yourself and make sure you have your life under control as much as possible.

- Do not sit back and let others look after you all the time.

How long will I be in hospital following bypass surgery?

A total of seven to eight days on average. Older people and more complex cases may be kept in a little longer.

Other treatments for angina

Most other treatments for angina have no scientifically proven benefit. That said, many people with angina do better with attention and encouragement.

Complementary therapies which encourage relaxation may be useful if you are stressed. In the 1930s it was shown that even *placebo* (inactive) tablets could be helpful, relieving pain in a third of people with angina. Any effects with unproven treatment may therefore be the results of the placebo effect. As long as complementary treatment – be it herbs, acupuncture or reflexology – does no harm, feel free to try it. Bear in mind that, if the treatments were really proven to be useful, all doctors would be recommending them!

People who recommend these treatments tend to deride the scepticism sometimes shown by doctors but, even so, often do not provide the proof of success or submit the therapy to scientific validation. If someone could prove to me that massaging your right big toe was safe and relieved angina, I'd be the first to recommend it. I would have to advise you on the evidence (called evidence-based medicine) and there is none so far. Lots of people started using beta carotene for heart disease and cancer. Proper clinical trials have shown no benefit for this but did raise anxieties about adverse effects (see the section on *Risks of high cholesterol levels* in Chapter 3). If you want to try an alternative approach, first be sure it is safe, then ask what proof there is. Always remember that isolated dramatic cases could be the result of the placebo factor.

I am not too sure what the 'placebo factor' means. Can you explain this to me?

Placebo translated from Latin means 'I will please'. A placebo effect is a benefit that cannot be explained by chemical actions from drugs or any scientific form of treatment. The benefit may be due to your belief (hope) that a treatment will work or just your total confidence in the doctor or alternative medicine practitioner ('This doctor is good; he will make me better'). Doctors use placebos to act as controls for their scientific preparations. Typically they will test a new drug for angina and compare it with a placebo in a way that you and your doctor do not know which preparation is being taken. This is known as a 'double blind trial' and is a means of making sure that a new drug really does convey a benefit.

Could alternative medicine with acupuncture, homeopathy or herbal therapy just be a placebo effect?

You have put your finger on the problem! Alternative therapies have not undergone the rigorous testing that doctors would like to see. However, it is difficult to study alternative therapies as there is little motivation from large drug companies to fund such studies, since herbs cannot be patented. Alternative medicine practitioners believe there is no need for this sort of study, as they feel the ideas have been practised for many years.

What types of alternative therapy are available for people with heart problems?

Acupuncture uses needles at various points of the body to release energy (*chi*) and this is believed to be essential to good health. *Homeopathy* uses minute quantities of substances which produce similar symptoms to those experienced by people with heart problems, in the belief that resistance will develop. *Herbalism* uses plant-based preparations (in an alcohol base) believed to restore good health. Herbal medicine is known as phytotherapy (plant therapy) and is quite separate from homeopathy.

I have heard that herbs can be helpful in heart disease and angina. Can you give me some advice?

Any alternative therapy (e. g. herbs) should not replace an accurate conventional diagnosis but only be tried once the diagnosis has been made and the safety of that treatment established. Some of the effects that have been claimed for herbs and other plants include:

- breakdown of plaques in arteries (alfalfa; garlic; hawthorn; mistletoe);
- relaxation (lemon balm; lily-of-the-valley; St John's wort; valerian);
- relief of anginal symptoms (pineapple);
- lowering of hypertension (bugle; hawthorn; mistletoe; skullcap; yarrow);
- relief of stress and anxiety (camomile; skullcap; St John's wort);
- circulation stimulation (cayenne, ginger; hawthorn)
- diuretic (dandelion; lily-of-the-valley; yarrow);
- antioxidant (garlic);
- lowering of cholesterol (ginger; motherwort; onion);
- reduction of clotting (gingko; onion);
- relief of palpitations (motherwort).

None of the claims for these herbs has reliably passed scientific scrutiny, yet a whole industry exists based on the assertions made. Only garlic has been studied in any depth and, whilst there seems to be some benefit, it should be considered a supplement not an alternative (see the question on garlic in

Chapter 9). In other words, don't stop your medication, which has been scientifically proved to help, but do try complementary treatments that can be bought in reputable chemists' shops if you want to, following the advice on the information leaflets.

You keep emphasizing the importance of going to reputable shops to buy herbal medicine. Isn't all the information we need on the label?

Not necessarily! A recent study looked at 30 different boxes of feverfew, used to help migraine and arthritis. Only two preparations contained any feverfew at all. The problem is that medications are rigorously checked but herb preparations are not regulated.

Are Chinese herbs the same as our herbal medicines and can they help?

Chinese herbal medicine is based on a different philosophy and uses different preparations and diagnostic techniques to those in the West, so it is considered a separate branch of herbal medicine. Again, many claims are made, but there is little scientific evidence available. When I studied one Chinese herb recommended for angina, compared to placebo all it did was to cause more headaches!

Are you in favour or against alternative methods of treatment?

If any treatment makes you feel better and does no harm, I cannot be against it. You must, however, have a full medical history and examination to make sure that nothing is being missed. Herbal medicine is slow-acting and best for chronic conditions, so it may help angina. Certain herbs in excess can lead to side effects – parsley in very large quantities can cause liver damage, celery and angelica can cause the skin to be sensitive to sunlight, and many other herbs can cause stomach upsets. Some are even poisonous! This means that you should go

only to a qualified herbalist who knows how to handle the herbs
and select the right ones for you. The same goes for homeopathy
and acupuncture – only go to accredited people. There are some
addresses in Appendix 2.

I thought alternative medicine practitioners were all trained. Isn't this so?

No. Anyone can set up as a specialist in complementary or
alternative medicine and there are no Government requirements
for training. This means that in the wrong hands, you could be
harmed or have a medical condition missed. Always check if the
practitioner is registered, has qualifications, is insured and is well
established in practice in the area.

Why are doctors so sceptical about alternative medicine?

Doctors, and for that matter nurses and other trained medical
people, have to qualify to certain standards and practise their
craft following strict guidelines and codes of ethics. They are
naturally suspicious of those who do not have to follow these
rigorous rules and can make claims which are not or cannot be
scientifically proven. Doctors are now being urged to practise
only 'evidence-based medicine' which is medicine absolutely
proven to be of benefit. They obviously wonder why others are
not strictly policed.

Do you think there is place then for alternative medicine or should I ignore it?

Yes there is a place for alternative medicine, provided that a full
medical assessment has been performed on you and that the
practitioner is fully qualified. Quality of life can be improved by
many things, including a placebo. Provided that there is no
evidence of harm, alternative treatments can be tried. There is no
evidence that alternative medicine will lengthen your life, so if
your life is threatened by heart disease, conventional medicine
will be essential for your protection.

Can complementary therapies do any harm?

The short answer is yes – so always go to your doctor if you are taking these products; if you have a heart condition, check before you try them. Here are some reported dangers:

- Ma huang (Ephedra) used for weight loss and energy enhancement may cause stroke, heart attacks and sudden death.

- Chelation has killed some patients.

- Siberian ginseng can falsely elevate digoxin drug levels, leading to incorrect decisions.

- Gingko inhibits clotting and may increase the effect of warfarin (ginger, garlic and ginseng do this also).

- St John's wort and gingko can deepen the effects of anaesthetics, cause blood pressure problems and bleeding. St John's wort can cause a fatal irregularity of the heart beat – avoid it!

I have read in the paper about laser surgery. This sounds exciting – is it being used everywhere?

The word laser sells newspapers and excites the reader. Laser balloons have come and gone because of a lack of benefit. The technique of transmyocardial laser revascularization (doctors like long names!) is a treatment using lasers to create tiny channels in the heart muscle from the inside. It can be done by opening the chest (surgically) or via the arteries, like a catheter procedure. Patients who are not suitable for angioplasty or bypass surgery can undergo this procedure, the idea being that blood from the inside of the ventricle (pump) feeds the muscle via the channels. The results vary a lot and it is still experimental; so, if this procedure is offered to you, make sure that there are no other options (if need be, get a second opinion), that the centre has ethical approval and a lot of experience. (There are cowboy doctors as well as cowboy builders!)

What drugs should I be on to help stop my angina problems coming back?

All patients with coronary disease should be taking:

- aspirin (or clopidogrel);

- a statin (dose increased to get LDL 2.6 mmol/litre or less);

- a beta-blocker (e.g. bisoprolol 5 mg or atenolol 50 mg daily). and

- an ACE inhibitor (e.g. perindopril up to 8 mg, ramipril 5–10 mg daily) or an AII inhibitor (e.g. valsartan, candesartan, losartan, irbesartan) providing there are no specific contraindications or side effects

If you are not on one of these drugs, ask why.

4
Heart attacks

The medical term for a heart attack is *myocardial infarction* (pronounced *myo-car-dee-al in-fark-shun*). The heart muscle is the myocardium; infarct means death – thus, death of heart muscle. Some people also use the term 'coronary' because the cause is a block of the coronary artery.

Every 30 seconds someone dies from coronary artery disease. It is the single most important cause of death for men and women. Coronary artery disease kills more people than all the cancers put together.

Will I be able to avoid a heart attack?

There is no guarantee (never say never!) but your risks can be lessened by heeding the following advice

- Do not smoke (not one cigarette, not at all).

- Avoid passive smoking (sit in non-smoking areas; if your family smokes, send them outside to do so!).

- Watch your blood pressure.

- Know your cholesterol level and keep it low by diet; and medication if necessary (this is very important).

- Eat plenty of fresh fruit and vegetables.

- Keep your weight down and take plenty of exercise.

- Enjoy alcohol in moderation.

Just as you service your car – service your body.

Can you tell me what causes a heart attack?

A heart attack occurs when an area of heart muscle is deprived of blood because of a blockage in a coronary artery. As the muscle no longer has oxygen to feed it, it begins to die, chemicals build up and pain is felt. The cause is usually a clot forming on an area of narrowing in an artery (see Chapter 2).

I have recently heard that heart attacks can be caused by exhaust pollution. Is this true?

Recently a statistical link has been reported between car exhaust pollution and heart attacks with those most at risk being pedestrians, cyclists and drivers. Links like this have been shown before (e. g. in railwaymen in fume-filled tunnels) but no medical proof exists that it causes a heart attack, and there could be other interpretations of the association. An association does not mean a cause and most links like this raise more questions than are resolved. It is of course interesting, but there is little we can do about it other than change our travel methods on a large scale.

Symptoms

What are the symptoms of a heart attack?

Almost always there is chest pain. It usually builds up to become severe. It lasts longer than half an hour and, unless treated, may go on for 4–6 hours or more. The pain is most often across your chest

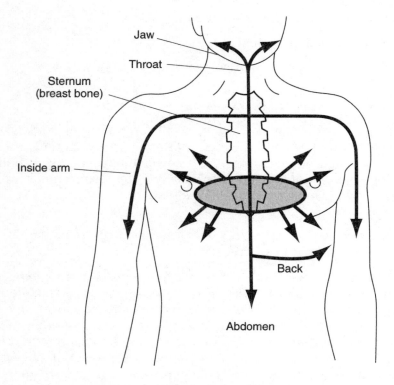

Figure 4.1 Site and radiation of heart pain.

and feels like a weight or a tightness. Some people describe it with a clenched fist as if the pressure or squeezing of the pain resembles the clenching of the fist. The pain is rarely sharp like a knife and cannot be pointed to by one finger as it is spread across the chest. The pain comes from the same place, even if you change your position from standing to sitting or lying down (Figure 4.1).

You may also get pain down your arms, usually the inside, to your wrists. The left arm is more often affected than the right. It can go to your jaw, throat, back or stomach. The pain may be severe, causing sweating, and be associated with feeling sick (nausea) or vomiting.

So, get help fast if you have:

- a heavy feeling – a feeling like a weight or pressure, or a squeezing feeling like a band in the chest – that lasts longer than 20 minutes and builds up (heart attack pain usually builds up rather than being maximal at its onset);

- pain from your chest, going to your neck, jaw or arms (left more common than right) and lasting longer than 20 minutes;

- pain (or discomfort) along with nausea, sweating, feeling faint or short of breath.

Are there any warning signs that might point to an impending heart attack?

Many people complain of 'indigestion' for some days or weeks beforehand. What they have been experiencing is angina.

It is quite common for people who have had a heart attack to say that they have been very tired in the previous 3–6 months. Some complain of breathlessness (the tightness across the chest has a breathless feeling about it) and dropping off to sleep watching TV. Others have noticed an increased tendency to snore and irritability - feeling 'out of sorts', 'just not themselves'.

A new warning sign is that of men complaining of difficulty getting an erection. The blood vessels to the penis do not function properly and can reflect problems with the blood vessels to the heart. Erection problems in men are caused by smoking, raised cholesterol, blood pressure or diabetes – exactly the same as for the coronary arteries!

Play safe and go to the doctor. If it is a friend or relative, do not take no for an answer – get them to see a doctor. If you think it is a heart attack, do not delay: for every one hour's delay, one life in every hundred will be lost – dial the emergency services (999 in the UK).

I know that I get angina and have learnt to recognize the symptoms. How will I recognize the difference between the pain of angina and that of a heart attack?

Angina is the result of a temporary shortage of oxygen available to the heart muscle and is usually caused by exercise (e. g. walking up a hill) or strong emotion (especially anger) (see Chapter 3). The pain is most often a tightness or a weight on your chest that may spread to your neck or arms. Anginal pain passes off when you stop or reduce exercise or when you take a nitrate tablet or spray. It does not last longer than half an hour.

The cause of angina is narrowing of the coronary arteries. Think of the artery as a three-lane motorway and angina as the result of two lanes being coned off. All the traffic will get through if people travel slow enough but, at high speeds, three lanes will only go into one if someone stops to give way. If no one gives way there will be a crash blocking the third lane. This is what happens in a heart attack. A clot forms on the narrowed part to block the artery totally. Narrow coronary arteries are often described as being hardened or furred-up.

My brother has had a heart attack – according to the hospital. He says that he did not feel it happening. I thought a heart attack was painful.

Some heart attacks can be so minor that they are barely noticed but others can be more severe. The severity depends on which part of the artery is affected. If you look at the diagram of the heart in Chapter 1 (Figure 1.1), you will see that there are two main arteries shown – the right and left. The left divides into two main trunks. These branch again and again into smaller branches or tubes (*vessels*), supplying blood to all of the heart muscle. A blockage in one of the tiny vessels means that only a very small part of the heart is deprived of blood. A blockage in a larger branch affects a much larger area of heart muscle. Because the blood can no longer get through and feed the heart and remove waste from the muscle, chemicals build up to produce pain, as if the heart had been bruised.

Heart attack – the event

My mother has been told that she is 'at high risk' of a heart attack. I am her carer and am worried about what to do if I think she is having a heart attack.

Your mother should rest completely in a comfortable position, preferably lying flat with her feet slightly raised. Make her avoid any exertion: if you are at home, the floor is best, not the bed if stairs are involved. Call the ambulance immediately (dial 999) and tell them that you think that your mother is having a heart attack. Make sure that you stay on the line long enough to tell them precisely where she is. If you know her doctor's name, contact the surgery immediately: the doctor may be able to start treatment before the ambulance arrives. If your mother has been given glyceryl trinitrate tablets or sprays for angina, then one or two tablets or sprays should be given; 300 mg aspirin should be chewed, or dissolved and swallowed, unless she is allergic to it or she has a recently (inside 1 month) proven stomach ulcer; if in doubt, give it anyway – the benefit is greater than the risk.

Why do we have to say 'heart attack' when calling an ambulance?

Some areas have specially equipped ambulances in order to give immediate care to coronary patients – these are known as 'coronary ambulances'. The staff – often paramedics – are coronary trained and can deal with the situation and its problems with a great deal of expertise and skill.

We live in the country and fortunately have a very good local hospital. However, it does not have a coronary care unit like the general hospital 40 minutes away. Our doctor has advised us to go to the coronary care unit in the event of my husband having a heart attack. Why?

In the early hours after a heart attack, the build-up of chemicals can irritate the heart and upset the electrical system that controls the heart beat. A very irregular rhythm known as *ventricular fibrillation* (VF) can occur. In effect, it is as if the heart has stopped; all that is happening is that the heart muscle (ventricle) is chaotically wriggling like a bag of worms (fibrillating), and there is no blood leaving the heart as a result. This can be corrected by prompt medical treatment so that normal heart beats can be restored. Prompt treatment means being in the hands of the experts in a coronary care unit who can keep an eye on your husband hour by hour until the risk settles, usually after 24 hours.

Coronary care units employ highly trained nurses who deal with pain, monitor the heart and supervise specific treatments designed to minimize complications and speed recovery.

My partner is very stubborn and simply refuses to go to hospital. He is getting on now and not strong. He has been a life-long smoker. I do not want to upset him by making him go to hospital if he had a heart attack. Would he be able to stay at home?

Some doctors believe it is safe for people to stay at home provided that suitable facilities and care are available. The danger period is usually within the first 12 hours; if this time has passed already and there are no problems, it is probably as safe to be at home. Older people like your partner may be happier at home also. Home care involves the family, district nurses and family doctor, and its quality will depend on their availability and workload. It is unwise to be at home alone following a heart attack. If the heart attack has just happened, it is better to be in hospital, where everything is immediately to hand. This applies to young and old people of both sexes. There is clear evidence that otherwise fit people in their 80s benefit from thrombolysis (clot buster medication) and angioplasty (balloon treatment) where needed – and that means going to hospital.

Going to hospital

My husband has heart problems and I am told that he is 'at risk'. If he had a heart attack, what actually happens after hospital admission?

If your husband has a heart attack at home, an assessment is usually made in the ambulance. He will then go to the hospital casualty department; some hospitals have a 'fast-track' system and he would go straight to the Coronary Care Unit (CCU).

The hospital doctor will take blood for enzymes. These are contents of the muscle cells which leak out when there is damage. They help the doctor determine the size of the attack. Another chemical test is that for troponin, which is very sensitive for identifying damage – doctors talk of trop positive (damage)or trop negative (no damage). A recording of the electrical activity of your husband's heart (ECG or EKG, see Chapter 3) will be taken at least once and will usually confirm the diagnosis and help localize the area of damage; eight out of 10 heart attacks show on the first ECG and it is after this that clot buster drugs or angioplasty are offered. A chest X-ray will be taken to see if there is any fluid in his lungs.

Your husband will probably be given medication (morphine) to relieve pain and limit complications. Tablets or injections may be used to reduce fluid in his lungs (diuretics) and stabilize his heart beats if there is any irregularity causing concern. There are three sorts of medications which are most often used (unless there are specific reasons why they should not be given) because they protect the heart, improve survival and reduce complications (see the section on **Treatment** in Chapter 3).

- *Aspirin* thins the blood to help prevent further clots. He will be able to take this in the soluble form, 75 mg/day, and will probably take it for the rest of his life.

- *Beta-blockers* are medications that slow the heart down and reduce blood pressure. They protect the heart from too much physical and mental stress. Because these medications can improve your husband's chances of survival up to 6 years after a heart attack, they will be probably be given for some years. Commonly used preparations are atenolol, bisoprolol, propranolol, metoprolol and timolol.

- *Angiotensin-converting enzyme inhibitors* or ACE inhibitors help some people survive. Fewer people on these medications have heart failure and they help reduce the heart's tendency to enlarge after a heart attack. Commonly used tablets are captopril, lisinopril, enalapril, ramipril and perindopril.

In the coronary care unit (CCU), rest is crucial to allow his heart to recover. Visiting by immediate family only should be brief as he will often tire easily. Young children can often be upset by the visit so care is needed if they come to see him. A brief visit to see that 'daddy' or 'mummy' is okay may benefit both child and parent, but the child must be fully prepared for the sight of the equipment, which can be daunting. It may be better if a nurse takes the child into the unit in a matter of fact way; this can reduce the natural tendency for the family to become emotional at a time of great stress.

In the CCU meals are light, as heavy meals can increase the heart's work by 20%, and rest is really what is needed. Your husband will find fluids, soups and salads are the easiest options.

As part of life in the CCU, there are routine ECGs, chest X-rays and blood tests, all designed to monitor his progress.

My husband has gone into a Coronary Care Unit. What will happen when he returns to the general ward?

Most people leave coronary care after 24–48 hours. Everyone is an individual, not a statistic, so some leave sooner than others. Once your husband is back on the general ward, a restful atmosphere is still essential and visitors should be restricted to avoid fatigue. Fear and ignorance are the biggest problems at this stage, so it is very important for him to fully understand what is going on. Questions need answers, so do not suffer in silence worrying about something. The key to your husband's recovery will be for him and his family to participate actively in the rehabilitation process. Do not keep any facts from his family and friends, as this leads to emotional charades at a time when maximum support is needed.

He will normally leave hospital after 7–10 days, but your husband may be kept in a little longer if his doctor thinks that he needs longer to recover. During the recovery period he will be encouraged to increase his exercise gradually and he will be given advice on how to live and eat healthily.

Just before discharge from hospital, or within 6 weeks of a heart attack, an exercise ECG on a treadmill will be arranged for him. This is designed to rule out any further heart trouble and allows the doctor and your husband to judge how well his recovery is progressing.

What drugs should a heart attack patient be taking on leaving hospital?

Drugs may be used to protect from further events and these are:

- aspirin or clopidogrel

- statins

- beta blockers

- ACE inhibitors or AII antagonists.

He should also be taking written information explaining what has happened and what to do next. An appointment with cardiac rehabilitation is strongly recommended. Specific drugs many be used to control symptoms, e.g. diuretics (water tablets) to relieve fluid retention and breathlessness. All heart attack patients should understand what the medication is for – if unsure, always ask.

Recovery period

I always thought that having a heart attack was the end of the story. Now you give me the good news that nearly everyone recovers nowadays. Is this true?

The short answer is not everybody recovers, but the good news is that most people do. Indeed most people make a complete recovery and only a small number are left with a disabling limitation, such as chest pain on effort (angina) or excessive breathlessness. We can help most people get back on their feet, but sadly a small number, less than one in 10 cases, have suffered too much damage even for all the modern technology to overcome.

A friend of mine had a heart attack recently and is still in hospital. She rang me to say that she was coming out soon. Will she be completely dependent and unable to look after herself? What can she do for herself after leaving hospital?

Don't panic! The danger period has passed but, of course, going home means a change of environment with no friendly nurses immediately to hand to provide security and reassurance. Not surprisingly, I expect that she will feel uncertain, anxious and depressed for a while.

It is important for her not to be alone for the first 2 weeks after discharge from hospital so, if she normally lives alone, it is best for her to stay with relatives or friends who can provide the necessary support and, of course, be there to talk to. The hospital should have ensured that her doctor knows she is coming home so that a visit can be arranged by either the family doctor or practice nurse, to see how she is getting on. This may be worth confirming with the doctor's surgery. Special cardiac liaison nurses do home visits in some localities, providing an important link between patient and their family, family doctor and hospital.

I had a heart attack over a month ago and I now feel completely better. I am frustrated that my doctor wants me to vegetate at home! When will I be allowed to lead a normal life again after my heart attack?

Most people are back to normal 6–8 weeks after a heart attack and back at work within 2–3 months. Some people take early retirement because a favourable financial package has been offered, and they are getting close to retirement age anyway. This makes good sense. Women who were working part-time are less likely to go back, as their work was invariably an additional job to their other commitments. Career women, however, can get back to work as successfully as men do: of those who want to work, 80–90% will do so. If your heart was badly damaged, your doctor may advise you not to work, and you will also need to take into account how demanding your job was.

If you do go back to work, make sure that you maintain a healthy lifestyle with plenty of exercise, an active social and leisure life, and a good night's sleep to help recharge your batteries.

What should I do to help my recovery after my heart attack?

There are several important aspects to helping the recovery and these include:

- making sure that you take your medication (and understanding why you have been given it) and taking it in the correct dose;
- losing weight if you are overweight;

- increasing physical activity sensibly;
- learning to relax and getting a good night's sleep, and
- avoiding cigarette smoking (active or passive).

I am on the mend after a heart attack – a nasty shock! How will I feel in myself when I return home?

After a heart attack it is common for both you and your family and friends to worry and be a bit fearful. The fears most people have are that:

- they might die;
- they will lose their sex life;
- they might have to give up work;
- they might have a physical disability.

They might also feel:

- angry about why it happened;
- guilty about not taking advice, and
- depressed that life, as you have known it, is finished and somehow you will be less of a person.

These feelings and fears are discussed more fully below. Most of them pass quickly as you make progress and recover, but it is always good to express any anxieties and worries to the hospital staff or your family doctor when you are home, because they can nearly always be explained and this will help you to overcome them.

Joining a rehabilitation programme is a very important means of coming to terms with what has happened and helping you to be positive about the future. Your spouse or partner is welcome to attend and the education, understanding and support provided soon restore your confidence, enabling you to return to a normal sex life and work.

Am I likely to get more chest pain after I have recovered from my heart attack?

Most people do not, but just a few do get angina. An exercise test will be organized for you and treatment arranged (see Chapter 3). Always tell your doctor if you get any pain. You don't have to put up with it – there are lots of things that your doctor will be able to do for you.

I am home from hospital after having had a heart attack. Will I need surgery or angioplasty in the future?

The first priority is to let your heart heal up. An exercise test may suggest that you have further problems and, if so, an angiogram will be arranged for you (see the section on *Tests* in Chapter 3). If you have serious further trouble, you may be advised to have surgery or angioplasty so that these problems do not get worse. It is better to prevent further heart attacks by changing your lifestyle and taking the right medicine and treatment.

Emotional problems after a heart attack

Will I be able to resume a normal sex life after a heart attack?

The answer is definitely yes! Questions about sexual and emotional problems are asked by anyone who has had any serious health upsets, not just people with heart problems. This is such an important issue that it is covered in more detail in Chapter 8.

Why do I feel so angry about what has happened to me?

'Why did this happen to me' and 'Why now' are common questions asked. Heart attacks can occur at any time, not at a convenient time; they are always inconvenient. If you feel angry and bitter about what has happened, you are likely to be short of patience and irritable. You may take these feelings out on close friends and family; this is understandable but they too will be suffering. Remember that being angry is a stage in your recovery process and it will pass. Sometimes it is a good idea to discuss these feelings with someone who is not so close to you as family – that is why it is such a good idea to join a cardiac rehabilitation programme.

I still feel very moody at times after my heart attack. Why is this?

You may feel up and down, day by day, as you come to terms with what has happened. Don't worry about these mood swings or feeling as if you have 'the blues' – focus on resting and being positive about the future. Don't bottle your feelings up – talk to someone close, your family doctor or practice nurse. These feelings are all quite normal.

I am the one who has had a heart attack, but I now feel fine, perhaps a bit low sometimes, but my children really blame themselves over what happened. Why do they feel guilty?

Your family has been through a traumatic time also – they have been afraid of losing you and have had to put a brave face on every day. Children often feel guilty – teenagers in particular – that in some way they may have caused your heart attack. Explain to them that, although the heart attack was sudden (they all are), what caused it took years to develop and they could not be to blame. Talk a lot, don't suffer in silence or let your family suffer in silence. As the Americans say, 'let it all hang out' or these bad feelings will fester and become destructive.

I'm really depressed after my heart attack, which is unusual for me as I am usually 'bubbly'. My doctor tells me that this is normal after a heart attack. How will I know if I am 'medically' depressed rather than just 'down'?

Being down in the dumps at times is common for 2–3 months after a heart attack but this will lessen as you get back to normal. Some people may have been inclined to be depressed before a heart attack, and this can develop into a more significant medical problem. Constant irritability and heavy drinking are early signs. Other problems include:

- difficulty in sleeping;
- lack of energy;
- poor appetite;
- loss of interest in your old activities ('I can't be bothered to go visiting');
- unable to concentrate ('I pick up the paper, put it down, pick it up, forget what I have just read');
- paying less attention to your appearance.

More serious cases are associated with a feeling of no value, being worthless and having thoughts of suicide.

You must make sure that your doctor is aware of these feelings, as medication or counselling can help the way you feel. There is no need to put up with feeling depressed nor for you and your family to suffer. If life seems desperate, phone the Samaritans or go to the hospital – seek help.

Treatment

What treatment will I be given when I leave hospital following my heart attack?

Some medication is prescribed as a matter of course because you will have a better chance of survival and complications can be prevented. Medication includes aspirin, beta-blockers and ACE inhibitors (see the section on *Treatment* in Chapter 3). Not all medicines suit everyone and not everyone needs them, but you should be aware if you are taking them and, if not, why not. For some reason, not all people are given the medication that they need: only one third of those people who should be on beta-blockers are prescribed them. Because you have a 25% better chance of survival if you are given beta-blockers, it is important to know why you haven't been given them. Ask you doctor why are you are not on them if you have not been prescribed these tablets.

Other tablets may be prescribed for specific problems, for example water pills (diuretics) to reduce fluid retention and help breathing, and special medication to regulate your heart rhythm if it has been upset by the heart attack.

Just as it is vitally important to know what you are being treated with, it is equally important not to discontinue any treatment without checking with the doctor first. Simply stopping medication is a dangerous policy, as you could suddenly get a rebound effect and risk another heart attack occurring If you have side effects, tell your doctor so that your medication can be changed to another type.

If you had a heart attack whilst taking medication for another condition, such as high blood pressure or high cholesterol, it is essential to check whether treatments for these are still needed – they usually will be.

My husband has angina and I am worried that he may not survive a heart attack. What can I do if he has one suddenly – and what should I tell his friends to do?

Quick action is needed by you or his friends, as the muscle will stop working permanently if left without oxygen for 6 hours. The quicker you act, the better the chances of survival: getting help within 1 hour is better than within 2. He will have the very best chances of survival if you get help within the first 4 hours following the start of pain.

There are medications that can be used to break down the clot and open up the artery again. These are known as 'clot buster drugs' and the medical term for breaking down the clot is *thrombolysis* (pronounced *throm-bo-lie-siss*). Aspirin helps break down clots as do streptokinase or tissue plasminogen activators (TPAs). As these medications thin the blood, they are not used when there is a risk of bleeding elsewhere, for example if someone has a stomach ulcer or has recently had surgery. If you think your husband has had a heart attack, and he is able, get him to crunch a 300 mg aspirin into small pieces and swallow it before the trip to hospital. Some pieces will be absorbed quickly through the lining of the mouth.

Clot buster drugs slightly increase the chances of a stroke, but this is offset by a major reduction (40%) in his chances of death from a heart attack. Streptokinase is much less expensive than TPA. TPA is slightly more effective within 4 hours of a heart attack. If he is given streptokinase, his body becomes sensitive to its effects, so it cannot be used again for at least 12 months, but TPA can be used as many times as is needed. People treated with these medications are given a card to carry with them for future reference.

Clot busters are not always successful but do work for seven out of 10 people with heart attacks.

Is there an alternative to 'clot buster' drugs for heart attacks?

Apart from letting nature take its course, *percutaneous transluminal coronary angioplasty* (PTCA) is the only alternative. This is a means of unblocking arteries with a balloon and squashing the narrowings out of the way (see the section on **Angioplasty** in Chapter 3 with Figure 3.5). PTCA can be performed if clot busters fail or the pain returns after the clot busters have been tried, if there is a reason why such medications cannot be used safely, or if you are admitted to a unit where angioplasty is routinely available. Angioplasty with a stent inserted is the most successful way of opening the blocked artery and limiting heart muscle damage.

We were so grateful that my brother did not die from his heart attack. Why do some but not others die from a heart attack?

Sometimes the attack is just too big for all the modern treatment to cope with, sometimes the treatment just doesn't work and sometimes it's left too late. No matter how clever we are, there is always going to be a bad luck factor, but advances have increased your chances of surviving from 76 to 93% over the last 10 years.

Helping yourself

Exercise

I have always hated exercise. Now that I have had a heart attack, and presumably should take things easy, my doctor tells me that I need to take more exercise. What exercise should I be doing?

Many people like you who have had a heart attack were not physically fit before their heart attack: perhaps, because of pressures of work, there was little time for sport or leisure activities. Exercise is very good for you, but it does need to be enjoyed rather than seen or felt as a punishment. Dynamic exercise, involving movement such as walking, swimming, cycling, jogging, tennis, dancing and golf, is the most helpful. Isometric exercise, such as weight-lifting or press-ups, is not beneficial and should be avoided. Exercise should be undertaken every day but it is not compulsory, so avoid wet, cold and windy weather – consider walking in a new enclosed shopping mall if you have one near you. An exercise bicycle is a way of keeping up exercise when the weather is bad, and boredom can be avoided by putting the bike in front of the TV set.

Walking is very good exercise and it is cheap and safe. There is no need to take up jogging, if you don't want to – just walk briskly. Swimming is also good for the heart. At first, always stay in your own depth and do not dive in. Gradually increase to swimming some lengths of the pool as slowly as you like, and then speeding up.

Exercise should be increased gradually as the weeks go by. Some people feel unable to do much at first, and may even be afraid of doing anything at all or going out alone. Going out with relatives or friends helps but joining a rehabilitation programme, if possible, is the best way of regaining confidence and getting the maximum benefit.

During your first 2 weeks at home, do slightly more exercise each day in terms of distance and time. There is no need to be afraid of going up stairs or going for a walk. A useful plan is to cancel the daily paper and walk to the newsagent to collect it. This is exercise with a purpose: you can stop for a chat, and you know how long it takes to walk the distance to the shop, so the time it takes can be reduced as you speed up and get fitter.

It is a good idea to chart your exercise and how you are doing over the weeks following your heart attack. You may be surprised at how much you can already do and how much improvement you are making.

By 6 weeks after your heart attack, you should be back to normal activity, or even better, because most people do not exercise enough normally. There is more information in Chapter 10.

How I should begin my exercises?

It is always important to warm up first. Do some bending and stretching, and then set off at a gradual pace, gently speeding up. At the end of the exercise, allow time to cool down. See Chapter 10 for more information.

You hear horror stories about the dangers of exercise, from slipping a disk to straining muscles, or even dropping dead! Are there any 'commandments' that I should be following?

- Never exercise until it hurts. If you begin to feel uncomfortable, stop immediately and rest.

- Don't be embarrassed to rest – it is your health that matters, not your image.

- Avoid exercise within 2 hours of a main meal. The output from your heart rises by 20% to cope with digestion, so exercising too soon could make you feel unwell.

- Don't exercise if you feel under the weather with a cold or 'flu, or when you feel 'too tired'.

Warning signs that you are doing too much include:

- pain in your chest

- breathlessness

- palpitations (see Chapter 6)

- faint feelings, or

- just not feeling 'right'.

Stop immediately, and next time reduce the amount of exercise you do, stepping up again a week later. If warning signs continue when you are exercising less, go and see your doctor.

I am recuperating from a severe heart attack. How can I tell when I am overdoing things?

It is best to join a local cardiac rehabilitation programme, and most hospitals have these now. If you have not been told about such a programme, ask your doctor if there is one near you – it is most likely to have been overlooked.

Ask your doctor or nurse to show you how to take your pulse (see Figure 10.2). It should be less than 100 beats per minute (bpm) before you start exercising, and not go faster than 200 bpm minus your age: so if you are aged 60, your heart rate should not exceed 140 bpm. If your heart rate (measured at your pulse) is consistently greater than 100 bpm before you start exercising, it is best to get the doctor to check you over to make sure that all is well. At first your heart rate will rise quickly on exercise, but it will rise more slowly as you get fitter. If the rate goes above your maximum target, slow down as this is a sign you are overdoing things : it is very easy to be too keen!

Is it really necessary to know my heart rate?

No, it's not essential but some people like it as a guide. It is quite in order to judge based on how you feel and are you breathing comfortably. The best exercise is a progressive programme with a gradual increase in exercise supervised or guided by a rehabilitation nurse or physiotherapist.

I can honestly say that I have never taken any exercise, but my doctor tells me that I need to do so if I do not want more heart problems. For how long should I exercise?

Only for about 15 minutes at first. Don't overdo things: gradually increase the time and build more exercise into your day:

- Can you climb two flights of stairs instead of using a lift?
- Do you really need the car or the bus for the half mile or kilometre to the shops?
- Can you park half a mile from the station or get off the bus a stop early, and then walk the rest of the way?

Ideally exercise should be built up to 30–40 minutes a day, five or more times a week.

How will exercise help me?

- Exercise improves your breathing and thus the supply of oxygen.

- It strengthens your heart's pumping action.

- As your fitness improves, your general well-being improves, along with greater self-confidence.

- Any bottled up stress tends to be released, relaxation and sleep will be improved, and overall lethargy and fatigue decreased.

- Exercise also helps you lose weight and improves your cholesterol levels.

Exercise is cheap – all that is needed is the will to do it and a good pair of shoes.

Diet

Should I be doing anything about what I eat?

There are two main things about your eating that can be improved: reducing your weight and lowering your fat intake (cholesterol). Both are important and usually related, although some thin people can have high cholesterol levels, and some fat people can have normal cholesterol levels. See the section on *Risks of high cholesterol levels* in Chapter 2, for more information about cholesterol and lipids, and what is involved.

I am absolutely miserable when I go on a slimming diet – it never works anyway. What is so wrong with being fat?

Being overweight throws a strain on your heart and causes your blood pressure to rise. Fat people are less mobile and have more pain in their bones and joints.

Losing weight sensibly (and not going on a 'crash' diet) will benefit your heart and help keep your blood pressure normal. If you are overweight, losing weight may also help reduce the fats in your body. There are guidelines for your ideal weight (see Appendix 4). Losing weight is about changing your lifestyle and the amount of food you eat. It is not about becoming obsessed with food or going on crash diets. See Chapter 9 for more information about losing weight.

Would it help if I saw a dietitian?

Yes. Dietitians are extremely good at explaining which foods are best to eat, and they know how to advise different ethnic groups with specific dietary requirements. Ask for an appointment at the hospital or at your doctor's surgery.

My cholesterol was checked 2 weeks after my heart attack. It had gone right down, but my hospital doctor did not seem as pleased as I was. Why not?

After a heart attack, the cholesterol level will fall and return to your normal level after about 6–8 weeks. If it is tested on the day that you are admitted for the heart attack, this will be accurate too. Cholesterol measurements taken after the first 24 hours and up to 2 months after a heart attack are unreliable, tend to be low and therefore falsely reassuring. Whatever your cholesterol was, you will be placed on a statin (forever!) as the benefits are overwhelming. Your response will be checked to make sure that the dose is correct and that the targets have been reached (see the section on *Risks of high cholesterol levels* in Chapter 2).

I have read a lot about what I should do, now that I am home after my heart attack, but there seems to be too much to do at once.

It may seem that way at first, but it is important that you change your lifestyle. Don't get obsessed by the need to change, tackle each point of the diet as suggested in Chapter 9, in a gradual way. Get the whole family into healthy eating – pick up any hints or tips from family and friends, or leaflets from your pharmacist.

Begin with the simple tasks of reducing sugar, switching puddings to fruit, snacking sensibly on fruit and not biscuits, and then gradually switching from saturated to unsaturated fats. See the section on *Risks of high cholesterol levels* in Chapter 2 and then read Chapter 9.

5
Heart failure

Heart failure occurs when the body's demands for energy are not supplied properly because of a weakness in the heart itself. Heart failure from damage to the heart muscle is common and, at present, 0.3% of the UK population is affected each year. However, it becomes more of a problem with increasing age, as it affects 8% of those over 65 years of age. Put another way, many thousands of people develop heart failure each year, and this represents 5% of acute emergency admissions to hospital. Because heart failure is common in elderly people, one of the reasons why we are seeing more cases of heart failure is the fact that people are living longer. In total up to 2% of the population actually suffers – roughly 1 million people in the UK. Each year 120 000 people are admitted to hospital with heart failure and stay on average 11 days. Heart failure costs the NHS over £300 million per year. Heart failure, if not treated, can significantly shorten life and reduce its quality but we now have means of helping people to live longer and feel better.

Causes

Are the causes of heart failure known?

Heart failure usually occurs because of a weakness of the heart muscle. The heart then doesn't pump as strongly as it should. The most common cause of damage to the muscle is a heart attack but it can also be due to:

- narrowing (hardening) of the coronary arteries;

- high blood pressure;

- narrow or leaking valves;

- a disease of the muscle itself (usually a virus) or cardiomyopathy – the muscle is affected directly not as a consequence of other problems such as high blood pressure;

- excess alcohol consumption over many years.

My daughter has been diagnosed as having cardiomyopathy – what is this condition?

Cardiomyopathy (pronounced *car-dee-oh-my-opathee*) is a disease of the heart muscle. The muscles may be too thick – this is known as hypertrophic cardiomyopathy (*hypertrophy* means thickening) – or too thin and too weak so that the heart enlarges and looks flabby (doctors often call this a 'saggy bag' heart). Both conditions can cause heart failure. The commonest is the weak heart and the medical term for this is *congestive cardiomyopathy*. Hypertrophic cardiomyopathy is usually inherited and can be the cause of sudden death in apparently fit young people. Although coronary disease can cause weakness of the heart muscle, the diagnosis of cardiomyopathy in your daughter's case is probably related to disease of the heart muscle in the presence of normal coronary arteries.

I have read of footballers and other sports people dropping dead from HOCM – what is this?

Hypertrophic cardiomyopathy (see above question) can cause so much thickening of the heart muscle that it obstructs the flow of blood leaving the heart. It then becomes Hypertrophic Obstructive Cardiomyopathy or HOCM. This obstruction is increased when physical exercise or strong emotion increases the heart rate. It can then block the flow of blood or cause the heart's electric system to become so irregular from lack of oxygen that the person collapses (we call this *syncope* – sudden loss of consciousness). Sadly this collapse can be out of the blue and fatal. If it can be detected earlier, treatments are available with medication to help prevent this happening. People with HOCM should be managed in specialized units to allow for optimal care, as it is not a straightforward condition.

How often do sports players collapse and die?

Hypertrophic cardiomyopathy affects one in 500 people and along with other very rare conditions, it is estimated that 0.2% of the athletic population may have a problem with the heart that could affect them at some time. Deaths during sports have been estimated at between one in 100 000 and one in 300 000 in young athletes. However, in older people, because of the increased chance of having coronary disease, the death rate varies from one in 15 000 for joggers to one in 50 000 for marathon runners. Dramatic and newsworthy death during sports is rare. Currently the Football Association is using some of its income from TV coverage to screen all young would-be football stars by ECG and echocardiography – a commendable approach to safety in the sport.

My husband has heart failure but the doctor says his heart is OK, he's just anaemic - how can this be?

The heart can fail because of other problems. If there isn't enough blood (anaemia or blood loss, e. g. after an accident), the heart will overwork until it fails, because there is so little blood to pump around. It may also fail if the thyroid gland is overactive (*thyrotoxicosis*) because an overactive thyroid gland drives the heart very fast and can cause it to go into atrial fibrillation (see Chapter 6). Basically the heart is OK and recovers when the conditions are treated.

If the heart valves are to blame for weakened muscle, can they be replaced?

Yes. An operation to replace defective heart valves is a successful way of relieving heart failure, providing the heart muscles (the 'pump') are not too severely damaged (see Chapter 7).

I have been told that I have heart failure. Is heart failure dangerous?

It can be if not treated properly. People with mild heart failure usually lead a normal life, but more severe cases will be restricted in what they can do. The weaker the heart, the greater the problem. The good news is that modern drugs, especially the ACE inhibitors (see *Treatment* below), can add many high quality years to the life of anyone with heart failure. If you have heart failure, ask your doctor about ACE inhibitors if you are not taking them – they are very important drugs, and can help you a lot.

Symptoms

What are the symptoms of heart failure?

When your heart does not pump enough blood around the body, fluid builds up because there is not enough energy to push the fluid through the kidneys into your bladder. The medical word for a build-up of fluid is *oedema* (pronounced *ee-dee-ma*). If the fluid builds up in your lungs, you become breathless, with a wheeze or a cough, and you may produce frothy sputum. If the fluid builds up around your ankles, they will swell up and you will be able to see indentations from your shoes or socks or from pressing your skin with a finger (be careful, it can be painful).

My partner has been diagnosed with heart failure but no one would guess on meeting her. However, she does get breathless at night. Why is this?

Fluid builds up in her lungs when she lies down and, if she is asleep, her defences are down. She may wake up with a suffocating feeling. This is helped by standing or sitting up, as this will take the pressure off her lungs. Some people open the window, feeling the need to gulp in fresh air, others walk around or go downstairs to make a cup of tea. If you can reassure her that all is well, this will help her to keep calm. Tell your doctor that this is happening as medication can help to relieve it.

I have heart failure and am worried that I will not be able to lead an active life.

Patients with minimal heart failure usually have no limitations to ordinary physical activity. Mild heart failure leads to breathlessness on walking a mile on the flat, one or two flights of stairs or a long incline. Moderate heart failure tends to cause symptoms more readily – walking half a mile on the flat or one flight of stairs leads to needing a rest. Severe heart failure causes breathlessness on minimal effort and even at rest. Everyone is different, so personal issues are usually best discussed with your doctor.

The good news is that we have treatments that can relieve or at least improve any symptoms so that a better exercise ability and quality of life can be enjoyed. People with more severe symptoms have to learn to adapt their lifestyle once all treatments have been tried and they still remain limited. If you are overweight, reducing your weight can help by taking some of the workload off the weakened heart pump.

You will probably be able to go on holiday and travel as usual, but make your plans more carefully to avoid rushing to catch aeroplanes or trains. Discuss with your doctor if you are planning long journeys while you are on water tablets (see *Treatment* below) as these may need adjusting – dehydration can be a problem on long flights.

Sexual activity doesn't usually present a problem and is not harmful. As in all forms of exercise, breathlessness might limit what you can manage, so take advice if this occurs (see Chapter 8). Some tablets can make you lose your sexual drive and, if this has happened, you should mention this to your doctor rather than accept it. Your doctor may be able to change your medication. Remember, don't suddenly stop taking your medication as this could be dangerous.

People often keep to themselves their worries and anxieties, Don't do this – most of your problems can be alleviated: don't be afraid to let the doctor know what's on your mind.

I had a heart attack recently. My cardiologist tells me that my heart has weakened and that I have now got heart failure. Will the symptoms be noticeable?

Your weight may go up from the retention of fluid (1 kg = 1 litre or 1 lb = 1 pint). Your doctor will monitor treatment by measuring your weight loss after you have been prescribed *diuretics* (these are pills to make you pass more water). There are other symptoms that you might notice:

- feeling tired and washed out;

- swollen ankles ('I can't get my usual shoes on');

- swollen tummy (so your clothing is tight); and

- on occasions, you may get a bit confused.

My doctor says I have a hibernating myocardium. What does he mean?

Your heart muscle looks weak and damaged but is capable of getting a lot of its power back; the damage is not irreversible. The heart is literally hibernating. If your heart only appears to be damaged, it may be possible to strengthen it by angioplasty or surgery. If that is possible, your quality of life and length of life will be greatly improved.

The doctor will check your heart to see what its strength is, either with an echocardiogram, perhaps a nuclear (thallium) scan, or a technique known as positron emission tomography (PET for short) (see the section below on *Tests*).

Should I discuss the diagnosis of heart failure with my family?

It is always important with any illness to discuss its effects with close family friends and, if appropriate, workmates. Having heart failure may limit you because of breathlessness, fatigue and weakness. Your family and friends will be worried about you – by bringing them into the picture they will be able to help and support you.

Tests

It is important to know the cause of heart failure because, if it is mechanical (such as a leaking valve), you will need a mechanical solution (a new valve). If it is heart muscle failure, you will need tablets. A high blood pressure will need urgent treatment. Investigations sort this out. Usually you will have an ECG (see Chapter 2), a chest X-ray, blood tests and an echocardiogram. These are all discussed below.

The doctor at the hospital told me that I have heart failure. For some reason, he told me to report back for a chest X-ray. Why do I need a chest X-ray for heart failure?

An X-ray picture of your chest will tell him about the size of your heart and its shape; this will help the doctor work out the cause of your heart failure. He will also get a picture of your lungs and whether there is any infection or fluid there.

You will be asked to stand in front of an X-ray plate, and then told to breathe in and hold your breath for a few seconds. As you hold your breath, the picture is taken. Holding your breath will prevent a blurred image occurring. The X-ray dose is very small and not in any way dangerous.

Why do I need blood tests for heart failure?

Your doctor will need to make sure that you are not anaemic, as this can make heart failure worse (see earlier question). Your kidney function will also be checked and any evidence of a congested liver looked for. Blood may also be taken to make sure that your thyroid gland is not under- or overactive. Any evidence of liver damage from alcohol will be monitored. Liver congestion which is not unusual in heart failure improves rapidly with treatment.

My sister is very concerned that she has been given an appointment to have an echocardiogram. What is this?

This is a painless simple test which tells us about the size of her heart, how well it is working, how strong the muscle is and how the valves are working. It is often used to assess the significance of a heart murmur and the size of a heart attack, to see if any clots are forming and to calculate the efficiency of the heart's muscle pump.

How is an echocardiogram performed?

The room (usually in a hospital but sometimes at your family doctor's) is usually darkened to allow the doctor or technician to see the screen. You may be asked to lie on your back or side. A special type of jelly is put on your chest and a probe applied to the jelly. The probe is moved over your chest. Ultrasound waves (it is not an X-ray being taken) are bounced off your heart and a picture of the heart's movements and structure made (Figure 5.1).

You are usually able to see what is happening and the pictures are stored on video which the doctor may show you. It usually takes 20 minutes and is painless with no side effects.

Doppler ultrasound is also used and this measures the blood flow. It makes a noise like a washing machine.

I have heard that some echocardiograms are done by the patient swallowing a tube. Is this true and, if so, what is happening here?

Yes, it is true. The reason is that your gullet is situated behind the heart, and a scan from the gullet (*oesophagus* pronounced *ee-sof-a-gus*) gives better pictures than one on the chest, when the probe has to steer round the lungs. This is known as *transoesophageal* (via your food pipe) *echocardiography* (TOE or TEE in America). It is done when we need specialized

Figure 5.1 Having an echocardiogram taken.

additional information, particularly on valve or clot problems. The tube is not large and is usually passed after you have been given relaxing medication and a local spray anaesthetic to the mouth. Some people do find it unpleasant but it is a very important test to help guide your treatment.

I have an appointment at the hospital for a nuclear scan. This sounds rather dangerous to me. Is it harmful and how is a nuclear scan done?

The radioactive levels are very low and not at all dangerous – you won't glow in the dark! A scanning machine takes pictures of your heart following an injection of a radioactive material (usually thallium) into a vein. If your heart is healthy, the thallium is absorbed and an even picture will be shown. If there is damage to your heart, the thallium will not be taken up well by the bits of your heart that are not working efficiently. If there is scar tissue from a heart attack, there will be a gap or a hole in the picture as no thallium will be taken up. If your heart is made to work hard by an exercise test or by the injection of a stimulant to speed it up, the thallium will not travel well to any areas where there is a poor blood supply (such as in that caused by coronary narrowing). When your heart rests between beats and the demand for blood falls, thallium can reach this area. In this way, the scanner can give a very accurate and useful picture to your doctor. First it shows a deficit, but then shows whether this deficit can be rectified. If the scanner shows a hole in the picture which does not improve, then it is likely that the muscle is dead and cannot be improved.

The hospital has written to me and told me that I need a test called a SPECT. What is this?

This is *single photon emission computed tomography*. It is a 3-D scanning system. You will lie on a table and the scanner rotates to take pictures from different angles, again helping to identify damaged muscle or muscle suffering from a lack of blood supply. It is a sophisticated test but simple to do –like a standard thallium scan but with bells on!

I have had test after test until I feel that I could not be tested further. I now have been summoned for a nuclear scan. When is nuclear scanning specifically helpful?

Nuclear scanning can be very useful for people with angina, after a heart attack and when there is heart failure. It is a means of trying to assess the importance of each narrowing present, and whether any good can be done by treatment. It is more expensive than an exercise test but useful when exercise tests cannot be done (e. g. if you have arthritis), or when specific information on your heart muscle is needed that a treadmill exercise test cannot provide.

My wife was told that she is going to have a PET scan. How is PET different from SPECT?

PET is *positron emission tomography* and this is a very specialized technique involving nuclear scanning, and it accurately tells us about blood flow and whether the heart muscle is hibernating or not. It is a very expensive test (over £1000) so is used only when really necessary. It can, however, identify where help might be possible when other tests have not been able to show what can done; so, used carefully, it represents value for money.

Treatment

I have been told that I have heart failure but was also informed that I will not need treatment for some time. Why not and, if I have to have treatment in the future, what might it consist of?

First of all, the tests will decide on the cause of your heart failure. A high blood pressure, coronary artery disease, severe lung damage, excess alcohol and problems with the valves are all possible causes. A leaking valve may be repaired or replaced; a narrow valve can be replaced or stretched by a large balloon (see

DRUGS FOR HEART FAILURE

Diuretics (water pills)
>   amiloride
>   bendrofluazide
>   bumetanide
>   frusemide
>   spironolactone

Angiotensin converting enzyme inhibitors
>   captopril
>   cilazapril
>   enalapril
>   fosinopril
>   lisinopril
>   perindopril
>   quinapril
>   ramipril
>   trandolapril

Digoxin

Nitrates
>   isosorbide dinitrate
>   isosorbide mononitrate

Beta-blockers
>   bisoprolol
>   carvedilol
>   metoprolol

Angiotensin II antagonists
>   candesartan
>   irbesartan
>   losartan
>   valsartan

Chapter 7), and a big scar from a heart attack, which causes the muscle to stretch (*aneurysm*, pronounced *ann-ure-ism*), can be cut out. Most of the time the problem is likely to involve the muscle pump and your treatment then is with tablets (see Box).

I have had an unpleasant jolt, having a heart attack. I suppose that I ignored the advice and warnings. Now I am determined not to lose control again. What can I do to help myself with my heart problem (my doctor says it's heart failure)?

The main thing is to guard against increasing the fluid build-up in your body (in your lungs or legs particularly). Therefore:

- Try to lose weight.
- Keep as active as you can.
- Avoid salty foods or adding salt at the table.
- Weigh yourself every day to check to see if you have put on weight which might be due to increased fluid.
- Take your medicine as directed.

If you find it harder to breathe, your ankles puff up, or you feel generally washed out, go and see your doctor. Don't let the fluid build up too much as it alters the absorption of some medications making treatment more difficult.

Medication

I have been prescribed diuretics. What are these?

Diuretics are commonly known as water tablets. They act to stimulate the kidney to get rid of the excess fluid which causes breathlessness and swollen ankles. Some tablets act quickly (e. g. frusemide, bumetanide): you will notice that you need to go to the toilet a lot over the first four hours or so after you have taken the tablet – this occurs every time you take the tablets but is usually over with by six hours. You need to plan when to take the tablets, so that you are not caught short. Some are milder and gentler (thiazides) than others and these help to spread the passing of water over a 10–12 hour period.

Most diuretics flush potassium out of the body and this may need to be replaced by tablets. Blood tests will help the doctor keep an eye on the chemicals in your blood. Doctors measure the 'urea and electrolytes' levels in a blood sample; these levels monitor your kidney function, potassium and sodium (you can remember them as 'electric lights').

How will I know if the diuretics are working?

You will be able to breathe better and your ankles will be less swollen. Your weight will go down as the fluid is urinated out. If your weight goes up, you will need more water pills but, if it drops too low, you may need them reducing, as you may have got rid of too much fluid.

Sometimes the tablets don't work and the drugs have to be temporarily given by an injection in a vein. This usually needs specialized treatment in a hospital. Once the fluid levels have been controlled, the tablets will be started again and this usually keeps the fluid at bay.

My doctor tells me that I need digoxin to help my heart. Why?

Digoxin is a tablet which in some people helps regulate an irregular heartbeat (*atrial fibrillation* – see Chapter 6) and makes the heart more efficient. It is also used to strengthen the heart muscle, giving it more pumping power. If the drug builds up too much in your blood, it can cause loss of appetite and nausea. Your doctor may check the level of digoxin in the blood with a blood test and adjust the dose to get the best effect without side effects.

My doctor has taken me off water tablets and put me on ACE inhibitors, which don't agree with me at all – they just make me cough all the time. Why?

ACE inhibitors stands for angiotensin-converting enzyme inhibitors. These are very important medicines that, in some people, increase their ability to exercise, as well as reducing breathlessness and fatigue. People will feel better on this medication and their life can be prolonged. Side effects are rare but occasionally people get a dry hacking cough. This is more common in women and Chinese people. If your cough is a problem (and is not due to fluid), ACE inhibitors can be switched to AII antagonists (see under treatment in the section on *Risks of high blood pressure* in Chapter 2) which have similar effects without producing the cough. Research studies show they are very effective drugs and may improve treatment by being prescribed in addition to ACE inhibitors as well as an alternative if ACE inhibitors cannot be tolerated. Studies with candesartan and valsartan have given impressive results, which are probably applicable to the other AII drugs.

Generally, doctors try to get everyone with heart failure to take ACE inhibitors if at all possible. ACE inhibitors are prescribed with diuretics and have the advantage of retaining the potassium that the diuretics wash out. They are quite often prescribed with diuretics and digoxin. Commonly used ACE inhibitors are captopril, enalapril, lisinopril, ramipril and perindopril.

It is likely that more people will be on ACE inhibitors or AII drugs either alone or in combination as the research suggests patients with mild failure do not develop a more severe condition and overall well-being is improved.

My wife has heart failure and gets very breathless. She was prescribed nitrates at her last visit to the doctor. What are these for?

Nitrate tablets (isosorbide mononitrate or dinitrate) are sometimes used to help breathlessness, particularly if heart failure and angina occur together. Although the treatment is effective, headaches can be a limiting side effect (see the section on **Treatment** in Chapter 3).

I have been prescribed warfarin. I thought this was rat poison! Why am I taking it?

Warfarin is a blood-thinning medicine and is used to prevent clot formation if your heart beat is irregular (*atrial fibrillation* – see Chapter 6) or if the echocardiogram shows something that might mean you may develop clots. Warfarin reacts with many medicines and alcohol, so make sure you get a list of these drugs from your doctor. Regular sensible alcohol intake should not be harmful as the reaction between warfarin and alcohol will be constant, but drinking in bouts or heavily is dangerous as it may not only disturb the warfarin control but further damage the heart. Heart failure *caused* by alcohol means that you will have to stop drinking alcohol completely – the heart may improve as a result.

The effects of warfarin need to be monitored with regular blood tests. The INR(International Normalized Ratio) is a test for measuring the thinness of blood – normal is 1. On warfarin, the INR should be between 2.0 and 3.0. In some people the INR varies a lot for no obvious reason and blood tests have to be frequent for accurate monitoring. When the blood is stable, the test may be monthly or less frequent.

Machines are available to allow you to test and monitor yourself at home.

Should I be taking aspirin? I have heard a lot about it in the media recently.

Aspirin may be used instead of warfarin, particularly in milder cases of heart failure or when the heart rhythm is regular (normal sinus rhythm, not atrial fibrillation) Doses vary according to the diagnosis from 75 to 300 mg daily. Aspirin can upset the stomach so you may prefer the soluble form in a glass of water or with food. Coated aspirin (e. g. Nu-seals) is available to help protect the stomach if regular soluble aspirin upsets you. Clopidogrel 75 mg daily is an alternative.

Can I take other medicines while I am on any of these heart failure tablets?

Other medicines may be used for specific problems. Ask your doctor or chemist if there is any chance of a reaction. Do not take arthritis pills without first discussing them with your doctor, as they can interact with heart failure medication. Some antacids contain salt so ask the chemist about the choices available.

Should I be taking beta-blockers?

In the past, the response would have been a firm no. Now research has shown that, once the failure has been controlled, beta-blockers may improve both symptoms and survival. Dosage is very low to start with under hospital supervision. When starting beta-blockers, you may not feel as good at first but, after a week or two, you should gradually feel better.

I have heart failure – can you tell me which drugs I should be taking and why?

Yes. The list below should help:

- **Diuretics (water pills)**. These reduce fluid and relieve breathlessness and ankle swelling.

- **ACE inhibitors**. Used to improve the heart's pumping efficacy and improve life expectancy.

- **Warfarin**. Used in atrial fibrillation to reduce clots.

- **Digoxin**. Used to control atrial fibrillation and, in some severe cases in normal sinus rhythm, to improve symptoms.

- **Beta-blockers**. Used to improve symptoms and survival.

- **AII antagonists**. Used in cases where ACE inhibitors cause a cough, and in combination.

- **Statins**. Used to reduce cholesterol when coronary disease is also present.

I recently read about spironolactone. Will this be given to me?

Spironolactone is an old diuretic (water pill). In a study of more severe cases, when it was added to diuretics, such as frusemide and ACE inhibitors, further improvement was noted. A problem arose in that the ACE inhibitors were used in lower doses than usually recommended, so we are unclear as to the exact benefit. If ACE inhibitors cannot be used or increased in dose because of side effects, spironolactone should certainly be considered.

Can I help monitor my heart failure at home?

The easiest way is to weigh yourself at the same time of day with no clothes on. It is best first thing before breakfast. If you gain 1 kg, i.e. 1 litre of fluid (2 pints), this points to the need to increase your diuretics. If you gain weight 2 days on the run, ask your doctor for advice. If you have been given a weight plan already, follow the instructions regarding extra diuretics (water pills). Your weight should return to the baseline – if it does not, visit your doctor.

Surgery

I have been diagnosed as having heart failure. Will I be able to have a heart transplant?

If your heart muscle is very weak and your activity remains very limited in spite of optimal medical treatment, transplantation is the best option available to give you a better quality and length of life. You must be aged less than 60 years and have a good social and psychological background, as you will need to be mentally strong and have support and help available. Some people will not be suitable because of other serious illnesses or problems.

What does a heart transplant involve?

If you have been placed on a waiting list, you must be available within 2–3 hours of being called because the donor heart can only be transplanted within 6 hours of the death of the donor. You will usually be given a beeper or mobile phone. The donor heart should be of the same blood group and match as yours, as well as matching your immune system. The race and sex of the donor and recipient do not matter but the size of the heart should be similar to yours, although it does not need to be exactly the same.

The operation is performed on the bypass machine. The diseased heart is removed by separating it from all the vessels connected to it but the back walls of the right and left atria are left in place. The new heart is then stitched onto the vessels and the atria, and the bypass is discontinued to allow the new heart to take over (Figure 5.2).

After the transplant, which is a straightforward procedure, you will stay in hospital for 2–3 weeks whilst drugs are used to suppress rejection of the new heart. Biopsies via a small catheter are taken from the heart to look for signs of rejection. This is a simple, painless procedure performed under a local anaesthetic and uses a vein in the neck. You will remain on drugs always to keep rejection at bay, and you need to watch your lifestyle carefully: hardening of the arteries in the new heart is a particular problem and is checked for at regular intervals by your transplant doctor. A transplant that is successful will transform your life. After 1 year, eight out of 10 patients will still be alive, and six out of 10 will live beyond 5 years.

I've heard about an operation to reduce the size of the heart by cutting out a piece of heart muscle. It is claimed to help heart failure. Should I consider this before a transplant?

This is an experimental operation. In many of the cases, a new mitral valve is also put in, so that it is difficult to sort out which part of the operation has been successful. It must remain a part of a careful research programme before it is widely used. We need

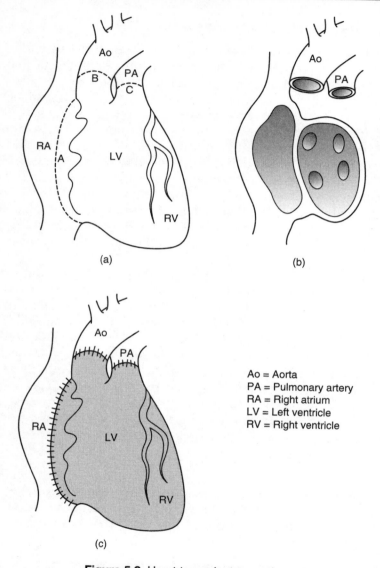

Figure 5.2 Heart transplant operation.
(a) Heart being removed, with cuts at A, B and C;
(b) no heart in place;
(c) new heart stitched on.

to know the risk of death at the time of the operation and if the operation works – for how long and what evidence there is for improved quality of life. It is still in its early phase of evaluation when caution should replace overenthusiasm.

My doctor has mentioned cardiomyoplasty but was not very enthusiastic about it. What is this operation?

This was an idea for surgery for the failing heart. A large muscle taken from a patient's back was loosened and then wrapped around the heart. A pacemaker was used to stimulate the muscle to squeeze the heart and give it more power. Initial enthusiasm has been replaced with disappointment as any benefit did not last long. It may have a place in certain rare inflammatory conditions which rule out a transplant.

Is an artificial heart another option for me?

It may be a short-term help, if the heart is severely inflamed by a virus, when it might buy time for recovery. It might also buy time for a transplant donor to be found. At present, it does not offer a long-term solution.

Can pacemakers be used to treat heart failure?

Pacemakers are usually used if there is an electrical fault with the heart (see the section on *How your heart works* in Chapter 1). However, a special pacing technique has been developed for heart failure, which can be used even if the electrical connections are intact. It is used in more severe cases and not everyone is suitable. Results have been very encouraging and it is certainly a treatment to consider.

6
Palpitations

The medical word for palpitations is *arrhythmia* (pronounced *ay-rith-mea*) meaning a change in the beating rhythm of the heart.

All of us feel the heart pounding away when we have to run for a bus, have seen an exciting film or had a fright: this is the normal response to exertion or excitement which causes the adrenaline in the blood to increase and stimulate the heart to beat faster. Being aware of the heart beat, when there is no obvious explanation, can be alarming and lead to anxiety and panic, all of which makes the situation worse.

What doctors mean by palpitations is an undue awareness of the heart beat. People see it in less matter of fact terms: 'missed beats', 'big beats', 'pounding', 'fluttering', 'as if my heart was going to jump out of my chest' are some of my patients' descriptions. Underlying these sensations the questions really bothering people are:

- Am I going to die?
- Will I have a heart attack?
- Will my heart stop beating?
- Will it damage me?

First, it is very rare for any form of palpitations to be dangerous or life-threatening. It is true that they are frightening and the fear can make them worse, but, for most people, all they have to fear is the fear, because palpitations do not usually mean disease.

For the vast majority of people, palpitations are just one of the ways that stresses and strains on the body show themselves, so they tend to be more common in people experiencing stress at home or work, in those with family anxieties and in those who are run down or overworked.

Types of palpitations

I often feel that my heart has missed a beat. Is this serious?

Missed beats are a common sort of palpitation and are invariably harmless. They can be brought on by too much caffeine, for example in tea, coffee, Coca-Cola or chocolate. Of these, coffee is by far the most important source of caffeine. Sometimes alcohol is the cause. If there is another disease present, missed beats may well be important, for example after a heart attack (see your doctor if you get these), but in nine out of 10 people the heart is sound.

I drink rather a lot of coffee. I have heard that caffeine is bad for the heart and I must admit that sometimes I feel that my heart has missed a beat. Am I about to have a heart attack?

The control of the heart is like an electric circuit with a master switch. Occasionally short circuits cause *extra beats* but the master switch is always in charge, even though it lets one or two extra beats escape. You may feel this more when your heart is slow, or when you are resting or just before going to sleep. It can also occur when the heart has been stimulated by caffeine, stress, or as a side effect of medication, such as inhalers for asthma. The extra beat arrives early and there is then a pause (the missed beat) whilst the next normal beat comes along. The extra beat may not be felt ('as if the heart skips a beat') but, after the pause, the pump of the heart will be fuller than usual, so the next normal beat will feel like a big beat – a 'kick' or a 'thump'. A beat hasn't really been missed, it just feels like it, and the big beat is the heart making up for the one that came a bit early. This is not dangerous – the heart is compensating for the early beat.

When I was at work the other day, I suddenly felt my heart was working overtime – I hadn't even been rushing up the stairs! What was happening?

Rapid palpitations may be normal, such as when you are running or excited, but sometimes they occur abruptly ('out of the blue') and can cause mainly fear, but also a sweaty feeling, light-headedness, breathlessness or, rarely, pain. Just as the cause of extra beats can be thought of as short circuits, so these palpitations are best thought of as caused by a sensitive area in the wiring of your heart. Again, it may be responding to stress, cigarettes, caffeine or alcohol. Remember that the wiring is only part of the building of the heart, a problem here or there is not going to affect the structure. However, palpitations which lead to chest pain, light-headedness or blackouts need a thorough medical check, so go to your doctor if you get these symptoms. Some people – a small number – have persistent troublesome rapid palpitations which carry on even when you have stopped drinking caffeine or alcohol or when you are no longer stressed. The cause can invariably be identified and treated and is rarely more than an awkward nuisance. Although there may be no major problem with the heart, there is no point in feeling ill if treatment can help you.

I've been very worried when I had two attacks of rapid heart beats recently. Are there any types of palpitations that are dangerous?

Some very rare palpitations are so fast that a blackout occurs. If they occur because your heart muscle is not working very well (*ventricular tachycardia* – tachycardia just means rapid heart beat), you will need medication to make them stop as they can be fatal. A common medication used is amiodarone. Your doctor will explain what is happening and it will be very important to follow his advice. You will need close hospital supervision. I must emphasize that this is rare.

I am in my twenties and am getting rapid heart beats every so often. I work in the type of job where results are all important. My husband has just lost his job as well, so sometimes I feel really stressed. Should I go to the doctor?

Rapid palpitations are a bit more of a problem because they are more scary. Again, younger people can be under stress, and the heart is behaving in an exaggerated variation of normal, as if you are running all the time, owing to higher adrenaline levels in the blood. A visit to your doctor and an ECG are necessary if symptoms are a problem (dizziness, breathlessness). The doctor will test you for various things such as anaemia, an overactive thyroid gland; he may also check to see whether you are pregnant, because pregnancy makes the heart beat faster in order to feed the baby. Very rarely, the ECG shows evidence of a specific 'extra wire' in the heart, which conducts beats much faster than the usual circuit; you will need to go to hospital in this case.

Self-help

I occasionally get palpitations. Now that I am approaching 50 are they going to get worse?

The first thing to do is not to panic. Your doctor will have already told you about not smoking and not drinking excess caffeine or alcohol. As you get older it is a good idea also to try and keep your weight down. Make sure that you:

- take your tablets regularly;

- attend your doctor for regular checks;

- report any change in how you feel.

I have just had three attacks of palpitations in a week, which made me very worried. By the time I got to see my doctor, they had gone away. What should I do if I get another attack?

When you experience palpitations, take deep breaths and try to relax. If you feel faint, sit down or lie down with your feet up. Try doing a deep cough. If the palpitations are missed beats or rapid beats, and you feel unwell or know that you have a heart condition, let your doctor know. If you are otherwise well and just afraid, look for factors that might have caused it:

- stress?

- caffeine?

- workload?

- alcohol?

- smoking?

- family anxiety or grief?

- problems at work?

- no recent holiday?

- generally run-down and anxious?

Try to help yourself by learning to relax more and avoid stimulants to the heart.

After you have tried the first-line principles of not panicking, taking deep breaths etc., try the following procedures, designed to stimulate a nerve called the *vagus nerve* which can switch palpitations off. These include:

- drinking ice-cold liquid or eating ice-cream, or putting your hand in a bucket of cold water;

- coughing deeply;

- blowing your nose with it pinched, as if trying to make your ears pop, for 20 seconds;

- pressing the right artery in the neck (this is known as *carotid sinus massage* (CSM) and needs medical instruction);

- **Do not press your eyes as this can be dangerous.**

If rapid palpitations are a more frequent problem or cause distressing symptoms, then medication will be needed to suppress them (see *Treatment* section below). Many types are available and more than one may be necessary. Just because you may need more than one medication does not mean that palpitations are dangerous, just awkward. Treatment is a bit hit and miss, so be patient and ask your doctor about any side effects.

I have heart disease and am finding that I occasionally get attacks of palpitations. Is this serious?

Missed beats in people with heart disease are not usually much to worry about but a check-up is a good idea. Those people on water pills (diuretics – see the question on diuretics in the section on *Risks of high blood pressure* in Chapter 2), or blood pressure pills (see Chapter 2) may have a low potassium level.

Although this is not a common cause of missed beats, the problem can easily be treated, so it should be considered if palpitations arise for no obvious reason when these medications are being taken. You should ask your doctor if your palpitations seem to arise for no apparent reason. Fresh fruit contains lots of potassium as does fruit juice, so the treatment is pleasant; however, it is best to avoid grapefruit juice as this affects the action of some medications.

There was something in the media about a problem with grapefruit juice interacting in some way with medications. Should I avoid the fruit or juice completely?

It is the concentrated juice that is a problem. The juice leaves the body via the liver where it shares the same breakdown system as some medications. It competes with the medications and stops them from being broken down (*metabolized*) so they may stay around much longer than normal and become more powerful.

I am in my sixties and have developed rapid heart beats in the last few weeks. I like to drink with friends most evenings. Do you think I am drinking too much?

Rapid palpitations in older people may be caused by atrial fibrillation (see below). This is an irregular heart beat caused by wear and tear but it is also more common in people with high blood pressure and those who drink a lot of alcohol. Sometimes it can be due to the coronary arteries becoming narrowed or to a thyroid problem (*thyrotoxicosis*).

If the rapid palpitations are other than normal speeding up (*sinus tachycardia*), your doctor may decide to treat you and base the treatment on how you feel. For instance, if your heart is sound and only one attack a month happens, then the main thing for you to do will be to cut down on your drinking which acts as a stimulant. Your doctor may treat you for high blood pressure.

I have tried all sorts of self-help methods but I keep getting attacks; when should I see the doctor?

Palpitations are common, mostly harmless but invariably worrying. Don't be afraid, try to understand the reasons – have a good look at how you are living and seek medical advice if there is not an obvious cause or the attacks just won't go away. If palpitations lead to symptoms of chest pain, light-headedness or blackouts, always get your doctor to check you over.

Tests

I have been to the doctor because I was so worried about these rapid heart beats that occurred. He has given me a little machine to record any attacks that I get in future. Can you tell me more about this please?

Because palpitations don't usually occur when you visit the doctor, a 24-hour ECG (see Chapter 2) is often used. This is like a 'Walkman' but it records your heart beats instead of playing music. The tape is replayed through a computer and we see the results in a matter of minutes. It does not record any sound so you need not worry that 'big brother' is listening in!

You can use this machine at home so that the doctors can watch what your heart is doing during normal daily life. You will be asked to keep a diary and the tape will be checked for times when you felt palpitations or became dizzy.

Four electrodes are attached to your chest and fastened with wires to the tape recorder which is worn on a belt round your waist (Figure 6.1). The monitor is quiet and you should not be inconvenienced.

Whilst using the recorder, act normally and try to bring on the symptoms you have been having. You are not allowed to have a bath or shower. You will be asked to return the recorder the next day so that we can analyse the tape and see if you need any

Figure 6.1 A mobile ECG recorder known as a Holter,
about the size of a 'Walkman'.

special treatment. Sometimes we do several recordings over two
to three days.

I think the machine that I am to be given is called a cardiomemo. Is this different to the 'Walkman'-type recorder?

This is a small machine which you put on your chest to record a
palpitation as it happens. It is about the size of a man's wallet and
can be carried easily. The palpitation is then decoded over the

telephone and printed out on an ECG. It is useful when attacks are infrequent but noticeable, and they have to be long enough for you to take action to record them. You will be shown how to use it by the technician at the outpatient department when you collect it.

There are now several recorders which you can activate yourself – some are very small so they are easy to live with. They store information which can then be downloaded and analysed on a computer. They are particularly useful when attacks are infrequent where a 24-hour ECG may miss them.

An appointment has been made for me to go to hospital for electrophysiological (EPS) tests. What are these?

These are tests which have to be done in hospital, not at home. Pacemaker catheters (usually four)are passed via a vein at the top of your leg to the heart and the source of palpitations pinpointed and analysed with complex computers. It usually takes up to an hour but can take a long time (several hours) and needs to be done with X-ray guidance in the catheter laboratory. The only pain you should feel is the local anaesthetic in the groin, but as the doctor moves the catheters you may become aware of your palpitations as the doctor identifies them and tries to get them to occur again. It is usually done as a day case, or one night in hospital may be advised.

Treatment

I have a very stressful job and find that I get really nervous. Is there anything that can help me?

Missed beats usually respond to self-help, perhaps with a doctor's reassurance which might include taking an ECG at rest and recording the heart beat for 24 hours (24-hour ECG see the *Tests* section above). A lot of people, who get palpitations like this, are young and under stress, and are helped by beta-blockers which block the stimulation of adrenaline and caffeine to the heart (see the question on beta-blockers in the section on *Risks of high blood pressure* in Chapter 2). These can be used for a month while you try and change your lifestyle where possible, and then as required, e. g. before a stressful meeting. Try not to drink too much coffee at meetings and change to decaffeinated-type drinks.

I am going for tests at the hospital next week for palpitations. Will I be offered any medication to treat irregular heart beats?

It will depend on what type of palpitations that you are found to have. There are a large number of medications used to slow down fast heart beats and to suppress extra beats.

- *Digoxin* (see *Treatment* section in Chapter 5) is most often used to control atrial fibrillation (see below). Doses vary according to how old you are and how good your kidneys are. Your body gets rid of digoxin through your kidneys so, if the kidney function is not as good as it should be, digoxin will build up in the blood. Commonest side effects are loss of appetite, nausea and vomiting. Your doctor may check the level of digoxin in the blood (6 hours after you have taken it) to make sure it is not too high or too low. If you get side effects, these will probably disappear if the dose is reduced.

- *Beta-blockers* (see under *Treatment* in the *Risks of high blood pressure* section in Chapter 2) are also used for controlling palpitations. They also help angina and blood pressure; they are especially useful if you have both of these conditions.

- The *calcium antagonists*, verapamil and diltiazem, are alternatives to beta-blockers for palpitations and, like beta-blockers, can be combined with digoxin.

Other more specific medications can be used to suppress extra beats and these include flecainide and amiodarone. These are powerful drugs, used if the simpler medications such as beta-blockers are not proving effective.

- *Flecainide* is effective in 30 minutes, so is often used as and when the attacks have to be stopped immediately. It is a very effective medication when taken on a regular daily basis by people whose lives are made a misery by troublesome palpitations, but it is unsafe to use it at all if you have heart failure or soon after a heart attack. It can cause nausea, dizziness, and unsteady feelings. Most people are quite happy on this treatment.

- *Amiodarone* is a life-saving medication for some but, because of its side effects, it is not normally used as a long-term treatment unless there is no alternative. It is very effective in the management of atrial fibrillation (see below), extra beats and dangerous palpitations, and it can be used when you have heart failure and after a heart attack. It takes some time to start working and can take a long time to leave the body. Side effects include sensitivity to sunlight, skin reactions, lung problems and disturbances of the thyroid gland and liver. You will need regular supervision so that the doctor can check for side effects. Amiodarone increases the action of warfarin so extra care is needed by your doctor to monitor the blood-thinning effects of warfarin, if you are taking this.

- Other drugs less frequently used and mainly alternatives to flecainide include *disopyramide, propafenone* and *mexiletene*. All are effective drugs but side effects can be a problem. If you are prescribed any of these drugs, always read the package label and discuss the potential benefits and side effects with your doctor.

Atrial fibrillation

I have just had a test for irregular heart beats and been told that I have atrial fibrillation. What is this?

Atrial fibrillation is a very specific irregular heart beat. The heart works like an electric circuit. There is a master switch at the top of the heart in one of the upper chambers – the *atria*, see Chapter 1. This switch regulates the speed of the heart beat and normally controls how and when the heart beats, by sending messages to the muscle pump (ventricle) which is located below the atria.

When the atria fibrillate (flutter), this means that the master switch is no longer in charge, discipline is gone and chaos reigns. Atrial fibrillation occurs at around 600 beats per minute (bpm) and the top chamber (atrium) resembles a wriggling bag of worms. The heart muscle (ventricle) could therefore, in theory, be bombarded with 600 bpm and would cease to work. Fortunately below the master switch there is a junction box (called the AV node) which prevents all 600 beats getting through to the heart muscle, so the heart beats at anything up to about 180 bpm, i. e. at the rate the junction box will allow. Medication is used to further block beats through this junction box so that the rate will settle to a more normal and pleasant 70–80 bpm. Doctors refer to the fibrillation being 'poorly controlled' or 'well controlled', depending on the rate achieved after medication. Good control is when the heart beats at less than 90–100 beats per minute.

Atrial fibrillation (or fluttering) is quite common and, for most people who get it, unavoidable. It responds to treatment and, although the heart is beating less efficiently than a normal regular heart rhythm, it can be improved, so that for most people it is hardly noticed. For a small number of people, it can be difficult to control and they will need to looked after carefully.

I have been diagnosed as having atrial fibrillation. What could have caused this?

It occurs in many conditions and, in a small number of people, for no obvious reason – so-called 'lone fibrillation'. It may be a part of getting older (wear and tear to the heart) but it can be a consequence of:

- mitral valve disease
- high blood pressure

- coronary heart disease
- heart failure
- an overactive thyroid gland.

Alcohol can cause atrial fibrillation in alcoholics but can also induce it in quite normal people when they have been celebrating a little too much, particularly in women, who are more sensitive to alcohol.

How will I know that the palpitations are due to atrial fibrillation?

Atrial fibrillation may come on suddenly and fast. It is usually felt as palpitations of a rapid sort, with the heart 'beating all over the place'. It can bring on chest pain but usually makes people breathless. Naturally it can be frightening, and may leave a feeling of light-headedness if it is so fast that the blood pressure drops a little.

Fibrillation in some people with heart failure can come and go and, as fibrillation is less efficient than normal rhythm ('sinus rhythm'), this can lead to periods of fatigue and breathlessness. For people who have atrial fibrillation regularly, it is important to keep the rate under control, or the efficiency of the heart and general well-being will be impaired.

My husband has just been told that he has atrial fibrillation. Is this dangerous and can anything be done to help him?

The short answer is: occasionally yes, it can be dangerous, but usually it is not. If he is given modern treatment, the efficiency of his heart will be improved, so that he will hardly notice that he has atrial fibrillation. If it comes on suddenly, he may become very breathless, and he may have to go into hospital. If he has an underlying heart problem, atrial fibrillation can cause little clots to form, and he will need blood thinning treatment to stop this, in order to reduce any chance of a stroke.

Tests for atrial fibrillation

**My doctor has told me that I have will have to undergo
some tests to check to see whether I have atrial
fibrillation? What will this involve?**

There are several diagnostic tests:

- Your heart may be checked by a standard resting ECG or
  one taken over 24 hours.
- A chest X-ray may be taken.
- A scan (echocardiogram) can be performed to check the
  heart valves and muscle pump (see the section on *Tests* in
  Chapter 3).
- Blood may be taken for routine checks and to make sure
  that your thyroid gland is all right.

In some cases, atrial fibrillation may be part of an illness which
needs surgery, e. g. mitral valve replacement (see Chapter 7), and
X-rays of the heart (cardiac catheterization – see Chapter 3) will
be performed before you have to undergo surgery.

You may undergo electrophysiological tests (EPS) studies (see
earlier question above) if you have rapid palpitations which
cannot be caught on tape, or if you have potentially dangerous
palpitations and have palpitations that refuse to respond to safe
and normally effective tablets. The reason for these studies is the
relatively new technique of cardiac ablation (see *Treatment of
atrial fibrillation* section below).

Treatment of atrial fibrillation

**What sort of treatment is there available for me now that
I have been diagnosed with atrial fibrillation. Can I just
be treated with medication?**

Following your test and depending on the severity of atrial
fibrillation, you will usually be prescribed medication, Those with

recent-onset atrial fibrillation may benefit from electric shock treatment.

If you have heart problems and the fibrillation is considered part of your illness, you will be treated with medication to keep your rate as steady as possible. To some extent your medication used will depend on the cause:

- If you have heart failure, you will be prescribed digoxin.
- If you have high blood pressure but no muscle pump damage, you may be prescribed a beta-blocker or verapamil.
- Once heart failure is controlled a beta-blocker may be added to digoxin or replace it.

Most people are on digoxin, but some are on more than one medication to get more benefit. It is vital that you know what each type is for (write it down when you are discussing it with your doctor) because, if you stop taking one medication, your heart may race away again. You will help yourself by reducing caffeine, alcohol, stopping smoking and reducing weight.

What medication will I offered to treat my atrial fibrillation?

Digoxin, beta-blockers (e. g. atenolol, bisoprolol, propranolol, metoprolol), calcium antagonists (e. g. verapamil, diltiazem), amiodarone, flecainide, propafenone, disopyramide, quinidine, and combinations of the above. Warfarin is used to thin your blood. See the section on *Medication* in Chapter 5.

I have been told that I am going to have shock treatment for atrial fibrillation. What will this involve and is it dangerous?

If the heart is all right and it appears to have been a temporary upset, you may undergo shock treatment to get the heart back to its regular rhythm.

Electric shock treatment involves passing a high voltage electric current through your heart and is known as *cardioversion* or a DC shock. It is used to correct rhythm disturbance, such as atrial fibrillation or rapid rates from an abnormal origin, and will

Figure 6.2 Electric shock treatment (cardioversion).

usually be performed if the fibrillation has been picked up early enough. The machine used is a defibrillator.

Under a brief general anaesthetic, an electric current is passed via a paddle on the top of your chest to a paddle on the left side or back(Figure 6.2). It takes less than five minutes. The abnormal palpitation is halted at its source, and this allows the normal electrics to take over. It is successful nine out of 10 times. Usually the patient receives warfarin for at least 2 weeks beforehand and a month afterwards to prevent the formation and dislodging of clots. If cardioversion is performed at short notice, your blood is thinned with heparin given through a vein. Cardioversion is usually done as a day-case procedure (in and out the same day) and you will notice how much better your heart behaves almost immediately.

There is no need to worry about electric shock treatment; it is safe and effective provided that all the precautions are taken – making sure of the diagnosis and use of warfarin.

A new technique involving a shock inside the heart is being used more frequently, as it appears to be more successful. A special tube is passed to the heart via the vein at the top of the leg under local anaesthetic. Once it is in place under heavy sedation or a brief general anaesthetic, a shock is delivered almost directly to the atrium, where the problem arises. The results are very encouraging, and you may be offered this as an alternative to the external shock treatment.

My cardiologist has mentioned cardiac ablation. What will this involve? Is it safe?

First, an electrophysiology study (EPS) is performed by a cardiologist in hospital(see the *Tests* section above). Once the source of the palpitation has been identified, and if the cardiologist considers you to be a suitable case, a special electrical pacemaker catheter can be placed at the source of the palpitations and radiofrequency waves used to ablate them (doctors often say 'zap'!). When the cardiologist is satisfied that all is well,all catheters are removed;pressure is applied to the vein at the top of the leg for 15 minutes or so, and after two to four hours' bed rest, you will be allowed up and about; you will usually go home the next day. An ECG will be taken to check the rhythm and a 24-hour ECG may be organized to judge the effectiveness of the procedure when you are out of hospital.

Cardiac ablation can be a lengthy procedure as the catheter has to be placed very accurately. It is usually successful and abolishes the palpitations, removing the need for medication. Very rarely, the normal electrics are damaged because the abnormal electrics are very close by and they can get caught by the ablation and a pacemaker is then needed.

The procedure can remove young people from a lifetime of dependence on medication; women can become pregnant without fear of any medication damaging the baby. Also, if medication is successful but gives side effects, cardiac ablation is an effective alternative. Because ablation is a *very* individual procedure, it is important to discuss fully with your cardiologist the potential risks and the chances of benefit for you – not someone in general, but you specifically.

Other abnormal heart beats

Two or three of my friends now have a pacemaker. Although I have 'funny' heart beats, I have not been offered one. When are they used?

Pacemakers will be used when the heart goes too slow. The heart can alternate between fast and slow; a pacemaker will still be needed as medication given to stop the heart beating too fast will make the slowing worse. A slow heart rate is known as a *bradycardia*. When the electrics of the heart fail to connect up, this is called *heart block*.

There seem to a lot of different methods of helping abnormal heart beats. Why was I offered electric shock treatment and not a pacemaker?

Shock treatment corrects a rapid abnormal heart beat whereas a pacemaker corrects a slow abnormal heart beat. If you have a mixture of fast and slow beats, you may need both treatments. If your heart occasionally speeds up, medication may be needed in addition to a pacemaker, to stop rapid palpitations or keep them under control.

I am going to have a pacemaker fitted next month – are there different types?

There are two types that your cardiologist will choose from, depending on which is most suitable for your problem:

- A temporary pacemaker (Figure 6.3a) will be needed sometimes after a heart attack if the electrics are bruised and a block occurs – it is fitted in an emergency.

- If the electrics are permanently slower or malfunctioning consistently, you will need a permanent pacemaker (Figures 6.3b,c). If you don't have this problem corrected, your body will lack oxygen and food; you will be tired and lethargic, and risk falling down from a blackout (see questions below). These pacemakers are small and very reliable computers which can identify your normal heart beats and the need to fill any gaps. You may need a permanent system if your heart does not recover when the temporary system is switched off or be advised that one is needed when you are seen in the outpatient clinic when it will be fitted electively.

I am rather nervous about having a pacemaker fitted. What will it involve?

For a permanent system, you will usually stay one night in hospital, although your hospital may undertake to fit the pacemaker as a day case. You will be told how long your stay is likely to be so that you can prepare a night bag if necessary.

For a *temporary* pacemaker, a wire is passed via a vein in the arm, neck or below your collar bone (most often) to the right ventricle (pumping chamber) and connected to a box at the bedside or attached to your arm (see Figure 6.3a). It is fitted under a local anaesthesia. This senses normal beats and fills any gaps with pacemaker beats. When the electrics recover, it is removed by simply pulling the wire out; this is not painful.

For a *permanent* pacemaker, you will be given a local anaesthetic and then one or two wires are passed to your heart via a vein under the collar bone (the subclavian vein), or the one running on the inside of your shoulder (cephalic vein). The pacemaker box is attached and buried under the skin. The wires are positioned with X-ray guidance and the procedure takes about one hour. A small cut is needed on the front of your chest below the collar bone and stitches will be used to close it up at the end of the procedure. Stitches that do not dissolve will be removed seven to ten days later, usually by the nurse at your doctor's surgery. Before you leave hospital, a chest X-ray will check that all is well, and the technician will use a magnet placed on the skin over the pacemaker box to make sure that it is working properly.

Before my heart started to play up, I was very active. Will I be able to go back to that sort of activity when I have had my pacemaker inserted?

The short answer is yes. A pacemaker is all about correcting a problem and allowing you to lead a normal active life. You will need the stitches out a week after the insertion and you will have been given a course of antibiotics to protect you from infection. You will not be allowed to drive a car for a week, and you must inform the DVLA and your car insurance company. You may be able to hold a Group II licence if there are no other disqualifying conditions, but you will need to wait 6 weeks. Group I licences are for motorcyclists, car and light goods vehicle drivers; group II relates to drivers of vehicles in excess of 3.5 metric tonnes laden weight, and bus or coach drivers. Group II standards apply to emergency police, firemen, ambulance drivers and taxi drivers.

You will given a check of your pacemaker function at 1 month and then once a year. This yearly check is to monitor its battery life. If the batteries begin to run down (many last over 10 years), the box will be unplugged from the wires and a new box implanted under local anaesthetic.

You will given a card to carry with you at all times. You will need to tell airport security as you will set off the alarms. Modern household microwaves and electricity do not affect it but mobile phones may do if placed close to the box (about 10 cm). Avoid placing them in shirt or jacket pockets on the pacemaker side. You will not be able to have an magnetic resonance imaging scan.

Life should not be restricted just because of a pacemaker.

Can pacemakers be troublesome?

Not usually, but occasionally they can cause soreness and, very rarely, become infected (it will then need to be removed). They may need adjusting from time to time – this is done via a computer placed over the box on the outside of the skin. Some early pacemakers developed faults and needed replacing. The wires in the heart do not usually displace after the first 24–48 hours. You can damage the wire or box in a heavy fall or accident,

Pacemaker out of skin and
into heart in a vein

Pacing box

Connecting wire

Enters skin below clavicle (collar bone) – part stays out
of skin and is connected by a wire to the pacing box

(a)

(c)

Electrode in
atrium

Electrode in ventricle

(b)

Figure 6.3 Pacemakers.
(**a**) Temporary pacemaker; (**b**) Permanent pacemaker;
(**c**) Permanent pacemaker in position.

and it should be checked if this happens. Contact sports should
be avoided (e.g. soccer, rugby). Most people have no problems at
all but, if you do have concerns, contact your pacemaker clinic
for advice.

When I went to see the cardiologist, he was very frank with me and said that the type of heart rhythm that I had was rather dangerous. He wants to insert an implantable defibrillator? Is this a type of pacemaker?

The official name for this is an *automatic implantable cardio-verter defibrillator* or AICD and, yes, it also acts as a pacemaker.

Some people have a very dangerous rhythm tendency which could cause them to drop dead suddenly. For people like you pacemaker wires are passed into the heart, under general or local anaesthetic, through the top of your chest wall through a big vein (*subclavian*) which runs under your collar bone. The defibrillator box is attached and then buried under the skin of your chest wall; sometimes it is placed in the abdomen in your stomach area. It recognizes normal beats but, if abnormal dangerous beats occur, it shocks your heart immediately. This may be felt as a slight thump. The machine needs checking at regular intervals to make sure that the battery life is satisfactory and, because it is a type of computer, it can also keep a check on how often it has been used. It is an expensive option but a definite lifesaver.

The British Heart Foundation book *Implantable cardioverter defibrillators* is a superb guide for patient and family (see Appendix 3).

A friend of mine has a defibrillator for atrial fibrillation – is this a new treatment?

Atrial defibrillators are relatively new. They are used in people who get very occasional attacks of atrial fibrillation – say two or three a year. They are inserted under local anaesthetic similar to a pacemaker, and provide a shock to correct the atrial fibrillation when an attack occurs.

Blackouts

My wife has suffered from blackouts recently. Can you tell me what these are and what causes them?

A blackout is a sudden loss of consciousness; this causes you to fall to the floor. If your wife's heart suddenly goes too fast or too slow, her blood pressure falls and she will collapse. It happens very suddenly; her colour drains away ('as white as a sheet'), but recovery is usually quick. You will probably notice that your wife's skin becomes flushed. Often she will recover so quickly that she may think that she has tripped up and 'wonder what the fuss was about'.

Sometimes it may be a faint, but blackouts can also be caused by lack of blood (anaemia), and problems with the nervous system (the brain), and a low blood sugar, e. g. in epilepsy or lack of blood from narrowed arteries. Blackouts from the heart problem tend to be sudden in onset with a quick recovery (5–10 minutes); blackouts *not* caused by a heart problem may be sudden in onset but recovery is slow, sometimes over several hours.

My wife has been ignoring these blackouts because they don't happen too often. Should I get her to go to the doctor and have these blackouts investigated?

Yes – she may need a pacemaker or medication to keep them under control.

How does a faint differ from a blackout?

Before a faint there is usually a warning. You may become pale and sweaty, yawn a lot and have a buzzing in your ears. Faints often occur in a warm close environment or when you have been standing for a long time in heat or a queue. A bad coughing bout can bring on a faint (*cough syncope*) and it can occur if men (and rarely women) get up suddenly at night to pass urine (*micturition syncope*). *Syncope* (pronounced *sin-co-pee*) is the medical word for a sudden loss of consciousness.

If my wife feels faint, what should I do to help?

Lay her down flat and raise her legs. As she recovers, gradually get her into the sitting position and then let her stand up. Make sure she is steady on her feet before she walks again.

7
Valve disease

This book is primarily about heart health and coronary artery disease. Sometimes heart valves become diseased, so a brief account of valve problems and their treatment is provided here.

The heart contains four valves which are designed to make sure that the blood flows one way only. Disease of the valves will distort the normal function of the heart. The two valves that are the most important are the mitral and aortic valves and these are the most commonly affected. Sometimes both can be affected at the same time. Each year 5000 people in the UK have valve surgery.

Two disorders can sometimes affect the aortic and mitral valves (see Chapter 1 for information on anatomy):

- they can leak (this is called *incompetence*);

- they can narrow (this is called *stenosis*).

The aortic valve normally has three flaps (leaflets) but some people are born with two and this causes early wear and tear. The normal three-leaflet valve may also harden up or become leaky with age. This can occur independently of coronary artery disease.

Causes

I have been diagnosed with valve disease. What do you think is likely to have caused it?

There are several causes of valve disease.

- Mitral stenosis (narrowing) can be caused by rheumatic fever. This condition, usually experienced in childhood or teens, can inflame the valves and lining of the heart, leaving permanent damage.

- Mitral incompetence (leaking) may be the result of rheumatic fever, bacterial infection (see below), a weakness of the valve supports causing the leaflets to flop backwards, or a narrowing of the coronary arteries.

- Aortic stenosis may be due to rheumatic fever, being born with an abnormal valve (congenital) or age (wear and tear).

- Aortic incompetence may be due to rheumatic fever, high blood pressure, bacterial infection, age and being born with an abnormal valve.

Symptoms

How will I recognize valvular disease?

If the aortic valve narrows, this can cause angina, breathlessness and blackouts, whereas, if it leaks, it usually causes the heart to enlarge and breathlessness then follows. If you feel tired and breathless on exertion, it is probably a good idea to go to the doctor for an opinion or tests. Valve disease may cause heart failure (see Chapter 5).

A severe mitral valve leak or narrowing will also cause breathlessness.

Both valves can become infected (see section on *Infection* below).

Does the fact that I have valve disease put a greater strain on my heart?

Yes. As a result of either narrowing or leaking or both, the abnormal valves increase the work that the heart has to do. If the valve is narrowed, the pump must generate higher and higher pressures to get the blood through. If the valve leaks, the pump must put out more blood with each beat: it must pump out the 5 litres that the body needs each minute plus the volume that has leaked back.

Tests

I have been asked to go for tests to see if I have valve disease. What will these involve?

The doctor can usually hear heart murmurs and will confirm the diagnosis with echocardiography (see Chapter 5). Sometimes a murmur is heard and a problem detected by chance. The echocardiogram provides a comprehensive picture of your heart, telling us about any valve leaks or narrowing and their severity. If your valve condition is not too bad, it can be watched by the echocardiogram at 12- or 6-monthly intervals. If the echo identifies a severe problem, you will be offered further investigations and possible surgery.

Treatment

Valve conditions that are not severe can initially be treated medically. Diuretics (water tablets – see Chapter 2) are used to relieve breathlessness; digoxin may be used if there is atrial fibrillation (Chapter 6), when warfarin will also be used. If the main problem is a leaky valve, ACE inhibitors (see Chapter 2) may be used to try to reduce the leak. They act to open up the arteries so that blood leaving the heart meets less resistance with the idea being to make it easier for blood to flow forwards rather than leak backwards.

I have had tests for valve disease and have been put on a waiting list for a new valve. What will this involve – it all sounds rather frightening.

Valve surgery is routine for the surgeon but a daunting experience for anyone about to undergo it! The surgeon should discuss with you the risks to you individually (if he doesn't, ask him) and explain what sort of valves are available and what the options are.

Preparation is similar to that for a coronary bypass operation (see Chapter 2). Your breast bone (*sternum*) will be cut along its length and your heart stopped; you will then be put on a bypass machine while your heart is being operated on. The surgeon will open up your heart to get access to the valves as these are located inside the heart. Sometimes a leaking mitral valve can be repaired and surgeons will do this if at all possible. Otherwise, an artificial valve is put in after the diseased valve has been cut out.

Your hospital stay will usually be 7–10 days. All heart surgery is a 'big operation' but we are lucky these days to have perfected the techniques and the risks are therefore minimized.

What will these artificial valves be like?

There are two sorts of valves used – tissue valves and mechanical valves. The decision as to which sort of valve to use will be made by the surgeon at the time of the operation because only then will a considered decision be able to be made – the surgeon will have explained the differences to you beforehand and you can indicate your preference should the surgeon have a choice when the operation is being performed.

- *Tissue valves* are made of natural tissue from humans, cows or pigs. They are treated to avoid rejection later.

- *Mechanical valves* are usually made of carbon fibre (but are often called metal or plastic valves) and contain no natural tissue. They may click.

A big difference between the two types is the need for warfarin, needed for ever if you receive a mechanical valve, whereas aspirin is all that will be needed if a tissue type is used (unless you are in atrial fibrillation).

How long do these valves last – is there a difference between these different types?

Mechanical valves last many years and rarely go wrong. Tissue valves can wear out after 10 years but the more modern ones last longer. Tissue valves are easier to live with but the chances of needing a repeat operation are higher.

It sounds like a big operation. What are my chances of pulling through?

Survival after a single valve replacement is 96%. There may be a slightly increased risk if coronary surgery is needed at the same time. This is more likely in older patients. Without an operation to replace a severely diseased valve, few people live beyond 2 years and quality of life is poor with a relentless downhill slide. Valve surgery will offer you an excellent chance of being alive and well 10 years on.

What happens if something goes wrong later. Can valve operations be repeated?

Yes. Repeat operations are generally safe to do and about 20% (one in five) need redoing after 10–15 years.

Do all diseased valves need an operation?

No, many minor problems never cause any concern. However, you will be checked regularly just in case these problems worsen. Even badly damaged valves need not be operated on straight away; the cardiologist will keep an eye on your condition and action will only being taken when symptoms become a problem.

Are there any other types of surgery for valve disease? I have been told there is something called 'balloon surgery'. What is this?

Leaking valves will need surgery. A narrow mitral valve, however, can be widened with a balloon. The decision to use a balloon depends on the appearance at transoesophageal echocardiography (see Chapter 3). If your case is suitable, a balloon operation on the mitral valve (*mitral valvuloplasty*) will be as successful as surgery.

Mitral valvuloplasty takes place in the cardiac catheter laboratory with a technique similar to coronary angioplasty (see Chapter 3).

Under local anaesthetic, the vein at the top of the leg is used. The vein goes into the right atrium which is separated from the left atrium by the atrial septum (see Chapter 1). The mitral valve lies between the left atrium and left ventricle, so the balloon needs to be in the left atrium in order to find its way through the valve. The septum is in the way, so a small hole is made in the atrial septum with a special needle which allows the cardiologist to position a large balloon behind and then through the valve. This method is necessary as the valve opens away from the cardiologist allowing the balloon to be passed forwards into the opening – the cardiologist more or less floats the balloon through as the valve opens with the blood flow. The balloon is blown up in the valve which is then split open along the flaps that have become stuck together. When the balloon and tubes are removed, the cardiologist will press on your groin over the vein to stop the bleeding. No stitches are used. If there are no complications, you will go home the next day.

Infection

I am about to undergo valve surgery. Are there any problems associated with valve replacement?

Heart valves can become infected and this is known as *bacterial endocarditis* (pronounced *en-doe-car-dye-tiss*). It can affect replacement valves and your own valves if they are diseased. Infection is not common but it is preventable. Your teeth and gums must be kept healthy: regular dental check-ups are needed. Bugs can enter the bloodstream via tooth decay while you are chewing. Any operative procedure that you undergo should be covered by a course of antibiotics to protect the valves – the medical term for this is *antibiotic prophylaxis*. Special antibiotic preparations are available on prescription.

Though rare, an infection that damages a valve is very dangerous and only half of infected people survive. As infection is preventable, this is one of those times when prevention really is life-saving.

I had a valve replacement some months ago. How will I know if I have developed an infection?

Infections develop slowly but you will increasingly notice these symptoms:

- raised temperature
- sweating at night time
- feeling more and more ill
- weight loss
- poor appetite
- joint aches and pains.

If you develop any of these symptoms, go straight to your doctor. If the doctor suspects endocarditis, he will send you straight to hospital.

When I was in hospital for a valve replacement, one of the patients there had developed an infection. Is infection common? Is it likely that I shall develop an infection too?

It is not common, but it is preventable. If it is caught early, 50% of people will recover. Therefore, you should always be aware of the possible problems and symptoms. If you develop any of the symptoms discussed above, go straight to your doctor. You can get a credit card-sized warning card from the British Heart Foundation (see Appendix 2).

8
Sex and the heart

Having heart disease does not mean the end of an enjoyable, satisfying sex life.

For anyone who was previously sexually active, failing to resume sexual enjoyment may cause unnecessary frustration, irritability and marital discord. This applies to men and women in heterosexual relationships and the gay community. It is a long-standing stable sexual relationship that is important and, if it existed before the heart problem was detected, it should continue afterwards. Casual sex may be more stressful to your heart and this is discussed in a question below.

A new relationship developing after heart disease has been diagnosed in one or both partners should not present problems providing it has none of the dangers of a casual encounter. Relationships based on trust, understanding and love are not casual, and as they develop, no undue stress is placed on the heart. Above all else, if you are involved in a loving new relationship, do not let your anatomical heart interfere with your emotional and happy heart!

Questions that you may feel are difficult to ask your doctor!

What happens to my heart when I am making love?

As you become aroused, your heart rate begins to increase and you breathe a little faster; as the excitement increases, both the heart rate and the blood pressure increase, reaching their peak at orgasm and settling back to resting levels after about three minutes' rest. The average duration of sex is 15 minutes and the heart is really only stressed for 3 minutes.

If the heart rate is increasing, is sex stressful to the heart?

Sex is just another form of exercise as far as the heart is concerned. We have already said (in Chapter 3) that angina pain can be brought on by exercise, so pain could occur during sex, but the important point is that sexual activity is no more stressful to the heart than other normal daily activities. In one study using tape recordings of the heart beats during sex, the heart rate averaged 120 beats per minute and was less than that often seen during other daily activities. In another study, the blood pressure rise was not found to be dangerous or exaggerated.

The stress to the heart during sex is the same as 4 minutes on a treadmill exercise ECG. If you can do more than 4 minutes on that, making love should be OK. If your partner needs to be reassured, ask the doctor to arrange for the exercise ECG test to be performed in the presence of your partner.

Is casual sex more stressful to the heart than with a partner in a long-term relationship?

Yes, casual sex can be more stressful. Long-standing relationships, where people are comfortable with each other, should present no problem, but a casual encounter can lead to a greater heart rate rise. This is not harmful to a normal heart, but if coronary disease is present, problems may occur. There may be an age mis-match (e. g. older man, younger woman) and the environment unfamiliar (e. g. a hotel room), following too much food and drink (e. g. casual sex at an office party). Playing away therefore can be risky.

You sometimes hear horror stories of people dying while they are making love. Are these stories true?

You can die at any time and this includes during sex! The risk during sex is very low indeed and no higher than during other normal daily activities. However, it may be significant that, of those who die or have a heart attack during sex, 75% are having extramarital sex – so the advice is, beware!

I had a heart attack recently. How soon can I start making love again?

After a heart attack, providing there were no complications, sexual activity can be resumed in 2–3 weeks. Ask your doctor and use a stairs, walking or treadmill test (see below) as your guide. The advice is the same whether the patient is male or female.

Sex is normal and not unduly stressful for couples with a long-standing relationship and should be enjoyed as much by those with heart disease as those without. As you recover from a heart attack and return to normal activities, you should be able to return to the normal activity of sex.

I am in my early fifties and have had a heart attack. Am I too old for sex?

Age is not a barrier and even those in their 70s or 80s, who were previously sexually active, should not be afraid of resuming normal relations.

Men may take longer getting an erection and women may worry they are less attractive and find vaginal lubrication a problem (see question below on K-Y jelly). Sex should not be rushed – we have road rage but we don't need sex rage! Take your time, enjoy the build-up and use lubricants if necessary. Age is a time for mature reflection and a few wrinkles here and there do not detract from the beauty of the person within.

I had heart surgery 3 weeks ago. My husband is keen to make love again. Can I resume lovemaking safely?

You can resume as soon as you feel able. Chest wall pain can be a problem particularly when you are positioned underneath your husband. Mutual foreplay without full sex can be a satisfying alternative and may be a good way to restart sexual activity, particularly if your chest wall gives you some pain. Alternatively, try the side-to-side position, or experiment to find a position that is comfortable to both of you (see below).

After angioplasty, you can resume sex within two to three days, depending on whether your groin is bruised or painful.

As a useful guide, the stress on the heart equates to walking briskly (in 10 seconds) up and down two flights of household stairs (13 steps each) or walking one mile on the flat in 20 minutes. If no pain or undue breathlessness occurs, then sex should be symptom free. If angina does occur during one of these tests, repeat it following sublingual nitrate tablets or spray. If nitrates are effective, they can be taken before sex. Indeed, as a side effect, there is some evidence that nitrates improve sexual pleasure. Nitrates should not be used if Viagra has been taken.

My partner has recently had heart surgery but has been given the all clear. Are some positions during lovemaking dangerous?

No, not within the bounds of common sense. The heart does not appear to be unduly stressed in any position as long as the relationship is long-standing. Casual sex can be more stressful to the heart (see question above). See the question below about different positions that may be helpful.

The coarse hair which grows back on your partner's chest, where it has been shaved, may be uncomfortable for you ('it feels like a hedgehog'), and a small soft cushion placed between you can help (the sort of size you get on aeroplanes).

Since I came back from hospital following a heart attack, I've had no interest in making love. It upsets my partner and frustrates him. What should I say to him?

Most people resume sex as frequently as before the heart attack or surgery but others are less active. Some people are afraid that sex may damage the heart, spoiling a previously enjoyable sex life. They are often influenced by what is called 'Hollywood sex', which is the movie portrayal of overenthusiastic sex; in real life, sex may not be such a grand performance, and the stress on the heart is therefore not exaggerated.

Anxiety and depression may decrease your desire but, as your condition improves, your desire usually returns. Because you have a heart problem, you are now more aware of the heart beating, whereas before it had never concerned you. It will increase during lovemaking but there is nothing to fear: do the stair or walking test again to reassure yourself (see above).

If you are depressed (which is not unusual) after your heart attack or surgery, it usually lifts quickly (90% of the time), but a small number of people will continue to feel depressed and this will reduce or remove any desire for sex. When you do make love (infrequently), it is not fulfilling. Do not accept this situation – you are not 'past it' – seek help from your doctor. Medication for depression – often for only a short time – is very effective and side effects are not usually a problem.

At first, it may be that just touching, holding and caressing without intercourse will help you slowly return to a full sex life.

I have been diagnosed with angina. Will heart disease affect my sex drive?

No. There are too many people who believe in myths like this. Some think that their sex life is all over when they get to 50. This should be the prime of life. In medical terms, you will be pleased to know that middle age extends to 70 years! Once your symptoms have been dealt with, you should be able to resume lovemaking.

My wife and I have always had a vigorous and adventurous love life. Now I am worried that I may get angina while I am making love. Is this likely?

Angina may occur and is best treated with sublingual nitrates beforehand. Keep nitrates by the bedside, and take an extra spray or tablet if angina occurs during sex. Rest for 5–10 minutes, then resume if you wish to. If prolonged pain occurs, it could be a heart attack (this is very unusual): if the pain persists after 30 minutes, seek medical help. If angina is of a severity to limit sexual activity on a regular basis, you should be considered for fuller investigation with a view to angioplasty or surgery.

Breathlessness during sex may respond to nitrates but, if heart failure is the problem, your partner will need to adopt a more active role, and different positions could be tried. If you don't usually lie underneath, try this less stressful position or sit in a chair with your partner astride, facing you.

To be honest, our love life wasn't up to much before the heart attack. Will it get worse?

If you were having sexual difficulties (such as lack of interest, poor satisfaction, or inability to sustain or develop an erection if you are male) before your heart problems, these will get worse. It is important to talk about these problems, either individually or together with the doctor or members of the rehabilitation team. Specific sexual counselling from trained counsellors may help.

I have heart failure and find that sex is too much effort. What can I do?

This is difficult because your heart's pumping action has been reduced. The ACE inhibitors improve the heart's output and may help (see Chapter 2). Ask your doctor about them if you have not been prescribed them. Water pills (diuretics) may cause impotence as a side effect but you should not stop taking these. It may be possible to reduce the dosage which can help. Unfortunately, if your breathing depends on taking diuretics, the dosage will not be reduced.

Heart failure patients may be unable to sustain a full sexual relationship but cuddling, caressing, close contact and even foreplay will still enable you to enjoy a satisfying relationship.

Let your partner do most of the physical work and try different positions. If you are male and find that you can't get an erection, ask about available treatments (see next questions).

I am taking medication for my heart problem. Can medication affect my sex life?

The most obvious side effect of medication is male impotence – now known as erectile dysfunction or ED. Sometimes sex drive or desire (known as *libido*) can be reduced. Women may experience problems with arousal, desire, orgasm or feel pain due to lubrication problems. Drugs can be a problem, but it is most often the condition itself that leads to the ED in men. If a prescribed drug causes sexual problems it will do so in the first 2-4 weeks of its use and an alternative would then be worth trying. The drugs most often linked to ED are the beta-blockers and diuretics. and in the female sex drive or interest can be affected by beta-blockers. Statins used to lower cholesterol also rarely cause sexual difficulties – mainly ED in the male.

Whilst these effects may be drug-induced, they may also be psychological or due to your heart problem itself. Whatever you do, don't stop your medication, as this may lead to more heart problems; equally, don't accept the situation. Talk to your doctor: this is not a time to be shy or 'British'. Ask your doctor whether the tablets might affect your sex life. The doctor will know what you are talking about. Changing medication or adjusting dosage may help. If you are feeling depressed, antidepressants may correct the problem. However, if ED or sexual dysfunction (such as poor female lubrication or lack of interest) continues, it should be evaluated further. You may be given hormones, and men may have their prostate checked. Get specialist advice.

Since being on blood pressure pills, my husband is having a problem getting an erection – is there a connection?

Yes. Blood pressure tablets can sometimes cause erection failure in men and may affect some women also. If this happens, your husband should tell his doctor because a change in medication could solve the problem. Impotence is more common with diuretics and beta-blockers and less likely with angiotensin II antagonists and doxazosin.

Everyone has heard about Viagra. My husband has a poor erection – will it help him?

Viagra is a truly wonderful drug, but it does not suit or help everyone with erection problems (known as erectile dysfunction or ED). In 8 out of 10 people it helps restore an erection in men. It is not an aphrodisiac, so the penis will still need normal stimulation to make Viagra work. Doses are 25, 50 and 100 mg, taken 1 hour before sexual foreplay, and its effects lasts for 4–6 hours. Heart patients may benefit from Viagra because heart disease, rather than the drugs used to treat it, is the most common cause of ED. Always get advice from your doctor and do not buy it on the Internet. It does not cause heart attacks (nor do other treatments), any more than might occur by chance. Before trying it, you should have a check-up at the doctor's, and you may be asked to do an exercise ECG. Viagra reacts with nitrates and nicorandil (see the section on *Treatment* in Chapter 3). Oral nitrates and nicorandil must be stopped for 1 week before Viagra is used, and the nitrate tablets under the tongue or spray should not be used for 12 hours before or after Viagra. Nitrates plus Viagra can cause a dangerous fall in blood pressure. Otherwise, Viagra is a very safe and effective treatment, providing you are guided medically – do not experiment without a medical opinion.

A friend of mine had a heart attack after taking Viagra – it seems dangerous to me. What do media reports say?

There is no increased risk of a heart attack from Viagra – in fact there were less cases when Viagra was compared with a placebo (where there was no active tablet taken).

Does the effect of Viagra wear off the more you use it?

No. After a year, 87 out of 100 men who benefited from it, still did so.

What happens if I get angina during sex after taking Viagra?

Do not use a nitrate tablet or spray at the same time. Stop your activity and sit or stand up. The pain should gradually settle. A glass of whisky or brandy might be helpful. Do not try again until you have discussed the event with your doctor.

Are there other heart drugs that may react with Viagra?

Currently you are advised not to be on nicorandil (a potassium channel activator) or nevibolol (a beta-blocker) until research has reported that it is safe to do so.

Nitrates help my angina but I would like to try Viagra – what should I do?

Nitrates are relatively weak angina drugs, and have no proven benefit in preventing heart attacks or sudden death. They are used only to help relieve pain and breathlessness. Alternatives exist, so you can ask for your medicine to be changed. For example, you could try felodipine or amlodipine as alternatives. Once the change has proved successful (two weeks should be enough time), you can then try Viagra. Your doctor may need to ask a specialist about this, but most people can manage without nitrates.

I have tried Viagra but it only partly works – how can I improve things?

First of all don't despair. Viagra does not always work first time you try it – indeed some people need seven or eight attempts before it 'kicks in'. If it is not effective at 50 mg, try the 100 mg tablet. Only one tablet a day is advised and it should be taken on an empty stomach, and no smoking or alcohol is advised. It begins to work in 30 minutes, is at its peak after 1 hour and gives you 'a window of opportunity' for 4–6 hours. Remember that you have to be stimulated for it to work.

Side effects are not common. Headache and flushing with occasional indigestion occur but are not usually severe enough to warrant stopping taking it.

I have heard of newer Viagra like drugs – are they any different?

There are two drugs that work the same way as Viagra – Levitra and Cialis. Their real names are sildenafil (Viagra), vardenafil (Levitra) and tadalafil (Cialis). They all work in the same way blocking an enzyme known as phosphodiesterase-5 (PDE5) which controls blood flow to the penis. Blocking PDE5 increases flow so an erection occurs.

Levitra is very like Viagra and works at 5, 10 or 20 mg and, like Viagra, it is not necessary to take it on an empty stomach to get the full effect by 1 hour. However, sex with a full stomach is not a good idea for heart patients. There are no direct comparisons with Viagra, so all we can say is that it is an alternative with no clear theoretical advantage.

Cialis is different in one way – it lasts longer. It is available as 10 or 20 mg equal to 50 or 100 mg of Viagra. It reaches its peak effect 2 hours after it is taken but may be active 36 hours later. It is not affected by food. Side effects are similar for all three drugs but muscle pains are more common with Cialis. Again, no direct comparisons are available and ED success rates are similar. Cialis may, for some, allow more spontaneity but nitrates or nicorandil cannot be used for 48 hours afterwards. If you think you can't have sex without the risk of angina, Viagra's shorter action will be better for you, but when your condition has been stabilized and well controlled you will probably be given the choice.

If tablets don't work do I have any other choices?

Indeed you do – do not give up in despair. No treatment for ED harms the heart, so if one is safe, so are the others. Injection therapy and vacuum pumps are highly effective but need specialized advice, so ask for a referral. Before giving up on the Viagra approach, make sure you have tried the top dose. If you cannot take Viagra because you are on nitrates or nicorandil and they cannot be stopped, then there are other choices available (see next questions).

A friend of mine said he used a tablet under the tongue – I can't remember its name but it wasn't a nitrate. Is this another choice?

He was trying Uprima (apomorphine). This acts via the brain to release stimulatory chemicals. It is fast acting and does not react with nitrates. It only works in very mild cases and has been generally disappointing. Doses are 2 or 3 mg and mild side effects include nausea, yawning, fainting and headache.

Can I mix medications?

You can but there is no safety information or clear research evidence of benefit. It is not recommended outside carefully controlled research studies.

All I hear about is men's problems – do women get sexual difficulties and can they be helped, with Viagra for example?

Women certainly have sexual difficulties – known as sexual dysfunction or SD. Research is being done to see if treatments will help. The real problem is that the problem in men with getting an erection is obvious, whereas women's problems are not. Most doctors are men and have not been asking the right questions! Lubrication after the menopause is discussed above. Some drugs appear to suppress libido (sex drive or interest) and affect orgasms. Heart disease may also affect sexual confidence, as well as be a cause of reducing sexual enjoyment. Viagra may help, but we lack proof, so it is currently not recommended for women. Guidance is not really very clear, but still mention any problems that you are having – although we do not have clear-cut recommendations, by applying basic medicine and common sense, we may be able to help. Unless women raise the problem, the medical profession will not be aware of its scale and progress will be slow in helping.

Can you give me some advice in preparing for sex since my heart attack?

When heart disease has been diagnosed, it is important to follow the lifestyle changes discussed in previous chapters, and particularly in Chapters 9 and 10. Improving exercise ability and losing weight will help sexual ability also. Practical advice to minimize the stress on the heart during sex is as follows:

- Avoid sex within two hours of a bath or a heavy meal. Taking a shower and eating a light salad will be better.

- Keep the bedroom and sheets warm. You could invest in an electric blanket if it is cold.

- Don't make love if you are tired at the end of the day. Wait until the morning when you are refreshed and relaxed.

- Avoid caffeine, smoking or alcohol before or after sex. Alcohol may raise expectations that you cannot fulfil and it certainly does not enhance your sex life!

- If you get angina, use your nitrate tablets before lovemaking (but not if you are using Viagra).

- Don't rush into it – take your time.

- Use K-Y jelly if necessary (see question below).

I have heard that K-Y jelly can be useful if lovemaking is a problem or painful. How safe is it to use?

K-Y jelly is a lubricant which can be particularly useful if your vagina is dry. This sometimes occurs after the menopause and can be a problem in patients with heart problems who naturally but unnecessarily feel reluctant or are afraid of resuming a normal sex life. K-Y jelly has no effect on the heart and is totally safe. It does not reduce the effectiveness of or damage condoms.

Where anal intercourse is practised, K-Y jelly is very helpful at reducing any physical trauma to the anus or penis, the pain of which occasionally causes palpitations (see question below).

Does oral or anal sex stress the heart?

Oral sex should not stress your heart, providing both you and your partner are comfortable with it.

There is some evidence that anal sex increases palpitations but this has not been proved in a secure long-standing homosexual relationship.

I have resumed sex after my bypass and there are no problems, but I'm afraid that it might do some damage to the operation site. Is this possible?

Firstly, it is good to know that you have returned to a normal sexual relationship – we would like all people undergoing heart surgery such as yours to achieve the same because it is safe and enjoyable. To answer your question directly – no, the operation cannot be damaged: stitches will not be torn and nothing will fall apart! It is important to remember that sex should be an enjoyable fulfilling experience whether there is heart disease or not – people with heart disease can enjoy a sexual relationship whatever their age.

9
Diet

There has been a lot of talk about diet, both in this book and in the media in general, about the importance of good, healthy eating to keep your heart in good shape. The questions below will answer, I hope, all the questions that you may have about food types, a healthy diet and losing weight. When we use the word 'diet' we do not mean crash diets to lose weight, but adopting a healthy lifestyle with balanced nutrition, which is far more important and safer.

In the past, many doctors have doubted the importance of lowering cholesterol and have in many ways hindered the management and prevention of coronary artery disease. We now have overwhelming evidence that a high cholesterol causes coronary disease, and that lowering it encourages heart health and prevents the consequences of coronary disease by reducing heart attacks and the need for surgery or angioplasty. Fears that lowering cholesterol simply meant that you died just as soon but from something else have been totally disprovedand the evidence accumulates daily to support the view that not only do people have less heart disease but they live better lives for longer. If you stop smoking, you will reduce your chances of lung cancer and heart disease; if you reduce your cholesterol you will reduce your chances of heart disease and stroke.

Eating healthily does not mean a boring diet. As the British Heart Foundation puts it 'Food should be fun' and can be healthy too. It's all about avoiding a premature death.

Food types and eating healthily

Fats

Fats or *lipids* are discussed fully in Chapter 2 in the section on **Risks of high cholesterol levels**. We discuss here what types of food are involved. Remember that fats are divided into saturated and unsaturated types and most foods contain a combination. The proportion varies depending on the food chosen.

Saturated fats are mainly of animal origin. They are usually hard at room temperature. They can also be found in some vegetable fats. Too much saturated fat can be bad for the heart and it is the saturated fat that raises cholesterol. They are found in:

- red meat
- butter/milk/cheese/cream
- suet and lard
- some vegetable fats, especially coconut and palm oil
- cakes/biscuits
- chocolate, and
- most puddings.

Unsaturated fats are mainly of vegetable origin. They are liquid or soft solids at room temperature. There are two types:

- *polyunsaturated*, found in sunflower oil, soft margarines labelled 'high in polyunsaturates'; these fats can lower cholesterol;

- *monounsaturates*, found in olive and rapeseed oil.

I have read that fish oil is very good for you. Can you tell me about this?

Oily fish contain a particular type of polyunsaturated fat (omega-3 fatty acid) and this has been shown to help prevent coronary disease partly by thinning the blood. Table 9.1 shows the healthiest fish to eat.

It is best to avoid potted prawns, rich fish pâtés and fish roe as these are rich in saturated fat. Shellfish such as:

- cockles, mussels, whelks

- shrimps, prawns, lobster

- squid

contain higher levels of cholesterol but are low in saturated fat and may therefore be eaten in moderation – once or twice a week.

Table 9.1 Content of omega-3 polyunsaturated fatty acids in oily fish

Oily fish	Omega-3 content (g per 100 g)
Mackerel	2.2
Herring	1.7
Sardines	1.7
Pilchards	1.7
Lake trout	1.6
Salmon	1.4
Halibut	0.9
Rainbow trout	0.6
Tuna (less if tinned)	0.5

Fish oils can also be taken in the form of capsules. Oily fish have a particularly good effect in reducing triglycerides (see Chapter 2 in the section on *Risks of high cholesterol levels*), but some capsule preparations are high in calories, so be careful to check the label. Because of this, they have been known to upset people with diabetes and reduce the success of watching your weight. It is best to get your fish oil the natural way by regularly eating fish.

Omacor, a fish oil preparation, in addition to its benefit of reducing triglycerides, may be beneficial after a heart attack if triglycerides are raised in spite of statin therapy. The recommended dose is 1 g daily with food.

If I eat fish twice a week, will it allow me to eat what I like for the rest of the week?

No. A recent review of the scientific evidence about eating fish to protect against coronary artery disease concluded that 'merely adding fish to a nutritionally adverse diet will not grant a population immunity from epidemic coronary heart disease.' Translated this means that, if you are eating poorly, simply adding fish won't do any good. Fish should be part of a low saturated fat diet – part of a healthy eating plan.

I'm not keen on fish – can I have fish oil capsules instead?

There is no evidence that fish oil capsules *on their own* have any protective effect, but they represent a 'better than nothing' alternative.

What is the difference between white fish and oily fish?

White fish includes cod, haddock, halibut, plaice and monkfish; oily fish includes herrings, kippers, mackerel, salmon, sardines, anchovies, trout and tuna. White fish are low in fat and this is good for the heart. Oily fish in addition contain a lot of omega-3 fatty acids as well as vitamins A and E, all of which may be good for the heart, so they have a greater potential benefit.

I quite like fish but it can be expensive. How much is recommended to eat each week?

The current recommendation is 300 g (12 oz) twice a week. The average intake in the UK is currently half this.

How do I know if the fish is fresh? I would hate to get food poisoning.

Fresh fish is usually refrigerated with ice before being sold but it can be frozen, then thawed, and sold as fresh. The law says it must be labelled as thawed because refreezing thawed fish is a source of bacteria. The safest way of buying or eating fish is to consume fresh fish within 24 hours of purchase or to cook frozen fish from frozen or immediately it has been thawed *for the first time.*

Fresh fish are usually stiff, the eyes are bright and not sunken, and the gills are red in colour. The skin should be shiny. Fillets should smell fresh (of the sea) and have firm moist flesh; white fillets look white and almost translucent in colour. If you are not sure, do not buy it and do not be convinced by the fishmonger as to its freshness unless you know him very well. Do not buy frozen fish which is not solid or has white patches or ice crystals on the skin. Frozen fish should not be thawed in water as it loses its texture, flavour and nutrients.

Independent fishmongers tend to know more about fish than supermarket fresh fish counter assistants.

Isn't it possible to keep fresh fish in the fridge for a week?

Most fridges in our homes are set at about 3°C and fish spoils quickly at this temperature, so eat it within 24 hours. Stored on ice (0°C) fresh fish may last a week.

What types of food have low or high levels of fat and cholesterol in them?

Foods high in total fat
- Fried food
- Whole milk, cream, high-fat cheeses (e. g. Cheddar)
- Fatty meat and meat products, such as sausages and pâté

Foods high in saturated fat
- Fatty meat and meat products
- Foods cooked in lard, butter or hard margarines
- Cakes and pastries made with butter and hard margarines
- Palm and coconut oil
- Fatty poultry (duck, goose); poultry with the skin on

Foods high in total and LDL (bad) cholesterol
- Egg yolks (eat only three to four eggs a week at the most)
- Liver and other organ meats (kidney, brain, heart, sweetbreads)
- Shellfish (but these are lower in saturated fat than most meats and poultry so are fine to eat in moderation – see the question above on fish oils)

Foods high in polyunsaturated fat
- Some nuts and seeds (e. g. chestnuts, walnuts, *not* coconut)
- Oily fish
- Many soft margarines and vegetable oils (check the labels)

Foods high in monounsaturated fat
- Olive oil and olives
- Rapeseed oil
- Margarines and spreads made from olive oil.

What sort of foods should I eat to cut down on my fat intake?

Basically, avoid full fat dairy produce, deep-fried foods, pastry, biscuits and puddings. See Table 9.2 for a comprehensive list of the healthiest foods to eat as regards fats, and those to eat in moderation, occasionally or best left alone. Don't panic – all the good things haven't been removed, it is just a modification as part of a new way of living.

For cutting down on dairy foods:

- Change whole milk dairy products to semiskimmed or skimmed.
- Change butter or hard margarine to poly- or monounsaturated margarine.
- Change lard or hard vegetable fats to pure vegetable oils (e. g. corn oil or olive oil, high in polyunsaturates and monounsaturates respectively) – but remember that all fats are high in calories.
- Change cream to low fat yoghurt or fromage frais.
- Change ice-cream to frozen yoghurt, sorbets or low fat frozen desserts.
- Change high fat cheeses (e. g. Cheddar, cream cheese) to lower fat cheeses (e. g. half fat Cheddar, Edam, Brie, Camembert, cottage cheese and lower fat soft cheese).

Eat no more than 170 g (6 oz) of cooked lean meat a day. If you do want to eat red meat:

- Eat the leaner cuts and always cut the fat off at the table.
- Avoid burgers, pork, meat pies, bacon and full fat sausages.
- Switch to chicken or turkey (but do not eat the skin).
- Switch to game meats instead of duck or goose which are fatty meats.
- Avoid processed meats (sausages, hot dogs, salami, pâté).
- Avoid high cholesterol organ meats (offal, such as liver, kidneys, sweetbreads).

Table 9.2 A guide to healthy eating*

Food types	Everyday foods
Cereals and breads	Flour and bread, pasta, breakfast cereals and porridge oats
Vegetables, fruit and pulses	Most kinds (fresh, dried, canned, frozen). Tofu and other soya products
Nuts	Nuts may be included in vegetarian diets to replace meats
Fish	Sardines, tuna, salmon, mackerel, trout, white fish (including haddock, cod, plaice) – steamed, grilled or baked, *not* fried
Meat	Chicken, turkey (both without skin), veal, lean ham
Eggs and dairy foods	Skimmed milk, cottage cheese, curd cheese, egg whites, low-fat yoghurt, low-fat fromage frais
Fats	All fats need to be limited
Preserves, spreads and sweets	Artificial sweeteners
Cakes, biscuits and desserts	Home-made cakes and biscuits made using low-fat recipes; jellies, sorbets, skimmed-milk puddings
Drinks	Tea, coffee, water, fruit juice, low-calorie soft drinks, clear soups
Other miscellaneous foods	Herbs, spices, mustard, vinegar, Worcester sauce, fat-free or low-fat salad dressings

* Information from *Trim the fat from your diet*, published by the British Heart Foundation

Eat in moderation	Eat with caution
Water biscuits; plain semi-sweet biscuits (e.g. rich tea, digestive) (once a week)	Fancy bread and pastries. (e.g croissants, brioches), cream crackers
Chips and roast potatoes cooked in oil marked *High in polyunsaturates* or olive oil (once a fortnight); avocados, olives, lower fat crisps (once a week)	Crisps, chips cooked in oil other than olive oil or oil marked *High in polyunsaturates*
Most nuts (use a few only) Most nuts (use a few only)	Coconut
Shellfish (e.g. lobster, crab, prawns)	Any fish in batter, fish roe (e.g. taramasalata)
Not more than 3 times a week: lean cuts of beef, pork, lamb, bacon, lean mince. Liver, kidney, meat paste	Visible fat on meat, sausages, pâté, duck, salami, meat pies and pasties, pork pies
Semi-skimmed milk; not more than 3 times a week: medium fat cheese (such as Edam, Brie, Camembert, Parmesan); half-fat cheeses (e.g. half-fat Cheddar); 3–4 eggs a week	Full-cream milk, cream cheese, most blue cheeses (e.g. Stilton), full fat yoghurt, condensed milk, cream, coffee creamers
Polyunsaturated margarines and oil (e.g. corn oil, sunflower oil, olive oil, low-fat spread)	Butter, dripping, lard, ghee, margarines not labelled *High in polyunsaturates*, blended vegetable oils
Jam, marmalade, honey, boiled sweets, fruit pastilles, sugar, peanut butter	Chocolates, toffees, fudge, mincemeat containing suet, chocolate spread
Occasional cakes, puddings and biscuits made with polyunsaturated margarine/oil (2–3 times a week), ice-cream	Ready-made cakes and biscuits, cream cakes, dairy cream ice-cream, full-fat milk puddings
Packet soups, alcohol, low-fat drinking chocolate and malted rinks	Cream soups, full-fat milk drinks and shakes, cream-based drinks
Low-calorie salad cream and mayonnaise, French dressing made with polyunsaturated or olive oil	Salad cream, mayonnaise, creamy dressings

- Cut down on egg yolks (no more than three or four per week) or consider the use of egg substitutes or egg whites in cooking.

- Eat fish that is low in saturated fat two or three times a week (you can include shellfish in moderation – see above). Try more oily fish than white fish.

- Avoid purchased baked goods like cakes (substitute bread or muffins – but check the label) or meat pies.

- Eat plenty of fresh fruit and vegetables (but avoid coconut, olives [not the oil] and avocados which are high in calories and may cause weight gain).

- Change from croissants to wholemeal bread.

- Substitute chestnuts or walnuts for peanuts, but remember that all nuts contain a lot of calories.

According to the TV ads, some margarines seems to be a good way of lowering cholesterol – do they really work?

Research has shown that Benecol, which contains special plant extracts, lowers cholesterol by 10–14%. Similar results are reported with Flora Pro-activ. Although these products lower cholesterol, there is no evidence that they reduce heart risk in the same way that statin drugs do (see the section on treatment under *Risks of high cholesterol levels* in Chapter 2). They are helpful when you have a borderline raised cholesterol, because you may be able to avoid drugs; but, if you have heart disease already, these products should be used with drugs – you will then benefit from the drugs, but the doses might be lowered. I do recommend them as part of healthy living, but price may be a problem for some people, and you will get benefits from supermarket spreads that are high in either poly- or monounsaturated fats, if the costs worry you.

My friend in America is taking nicotinic acid for her cholesterol – is it available here?

Nicotinic acid is available but not often used because of its side effects, especially flushing. It can also affect the liver and make any stomach ulcers worse. It can react with alcohol and upset control in people with diabetes, so doctors have to monitor anyone on this drug very carefully. Occasionally, It can make angina pain worse.

A new formulation (Niaspan) has just been launched. Nicotinic acid raises the good cholesterol (HDL) by up to 24%. Doctors will probably try it in those who have a low HDL in spite of being on statins, and therefore it is given in combination with these. Treatment will be introduced carefully and the dose gradually increased. Niaspan claims to cause less flushing than other types. Typical doses are 375, 500, 750 and 1000 mg, twice a day.

Someone told me that nuts were good for reducing coronary disease – should I eat them regularly?

Nuts (not coconut), eaten regularly (four times a week), have been linked to a reduction in heart attacks. Walnuts and almonds lower cholesterol. Therefore, nuts as part of a healthy lifestyle may reduce the risk of heart disease. Eat them with cereals, as a snack, or with a salad. Beware of added salt and remember that they have a high calorie content. If you use nuts in cooking, remember some visitors may be allergic to them.

Are there better ways of cooking I could try?

- Yes, grilling, barbecuing, braising, poaching, steaming, stir-frying or sautéing with minimal fat; baking, casseroling or microwaving instead of frying or roasting are better ways to reduce use of fats.

- Grill on a rack so that the fat drips away.

- If you have a roast, don't cook the meat in its own juice or make gravy from the juices. Cook the joint on a roasting rack and baste the meat with vegetable oil., lemon juice or a little olive oil.

- If you use a polyunsaturated margarine or oil for cooking, use as little as possible. Oil sprays are a way of avoiding excess in cooking.

Fibre

The doctor often recommends that I should eat more fibre. Is fibre important in my diet?

Fibre also means roughage. Most people associate roughage with bran but there are many foods which serve the same purpose (see Table 9.3). Starchy foods have the advantage that they are

Table 9.3 Foods and fibre content

High fibre foods	Low fibre foods
Wholegrain cereals (branflakes, muesli, porridge, wheat biscuits)	Plain and frosted rice cereals, cornflakes, Special K
Breads (wholewheat, granary, rye, wholewheat pitta)	White bread and rolls
Brown rice, pearl barley, bulgur wheat	White rice
Pasta (wholewheat)	Pasta (white)
Wholewheat crispbread, crisprolls	White biscuits and crackers (water biscuits)
Popcorn, Twiglets, wholewheat breadsticks	Cheese Puffs, Hula Hoops, pretzels, Quavers
Wholewheat and oatmeal biscuits (especially with dried fruit)	Rich tea biscuits, shortbread, wafers
Wholemeal scones, fruited teabreads	Pastries, cakes

filling without providing a lot of calories. Fibre passes through the bowel without being absorbed into your body and lowers cholesterol by reducing fatty foods in your diet. This type of fibre, known as soluble fibre (see question below), is effective in lowering cholesterol, if enough is eaten. It binds with bile salts from the liver, which are full of cholesterol, and prevents them from being absorbed. At the same time, by acting like a sponge absorbing water, it gives a full-up feeling. Soluble fibre-rich foods include

- pulse vegetables, such as peas, beans and lentils;

- fruit, such as bananas, apples, berries and citrus fruits; and

- oat cereals (not wheat).

The average person eats 15–20 g of fibre a day and this needs to be increased to over 25 g. As fibre is increased in the diet, it becomes important to drink plenty of fluids so that the swelling action can be achieved. Increase the fibre content gradually to give your digestive system a chance to adjust.

What is the difference between soluble and insoluble fibre. Should I eat both?

Insoluble fibre is important for digestion and taking it with fluid helps to prevent constipation and other bowel problems. Soluble fibre helps to lower cholesterol. Insoluble fibre is found in wholegrain and wholemeal foods (wholemeal bread, granary bread, brown rice, wholemeal or wholegrain flour and whole-wheat breakfast cereals). A mixed diet of both types of fibre will keep you regular and lower your cholesterol.

When I am in the supermarket, I get confused as to which foods are best for fibre content. Can you tell me more about which contain more fibre?

To increase fibre is not difficult. Aim to eat two items from this list each meal time:

- wholemeal bread or wholemeal chapatis or pitta bread;

- wholegrain cereal (bran, Weetabix, Shredded Wheat, porridge);

- baked potatoes (and eat the skins) instead of fried;

- wholegrain pasta and brown rice;

- fruit (particularly apples, pears, bananas) – fruit is also low in calories and rich in vitamins and antioxidants (see section on *Risks of high cholesterol levels* in Chapter 2);

- dried fruit, e. g. raisins;

- vegetables (particularly root vegetables such as carrots, turnips, parsnips; and green vegetables, such as sprouts cabbage, broccoli) – vegetables are also low in calories and rich in vitamins and antioxidants (see section on *Risks of high cholesterol levels* in Chapter 2);

- pulses, e. g. peas, beans, lentils, sweetcorn, baked beans, chickpeas;

- nuts, e. g. walnuts, chestnuts (but be careful, all nuts have a high calorie content).

Try to use wholemeal flour rather than white when you are baking, or a mixture of both. Table 9.3 gives a list of high versus low fibre foods.

I know that vegetables are good for me because they contain fibre and vitamins. I have heard that boiling vegetables loses the vitamins. How should I prepare fruit and vegetables to get the maximum benefits from them?

Many vitamins are lost in storage and on exposure to oxygen (air). Buy little and often and prepare just before you eat them. Leave the skin on where possible. Eat vegetables raw, or by steaming, stir-frying or microwaving. If you boil your vegetables, boil quickly in the minimum of water in a tightly covered pan and serve immediately. Use the cooking water for stock or gravy. Frozen vegetables are just as good as fresh and can be quick to prepare, convenient and economical. Dried fruits are high in calories.

Sugar

I have rather a sweet tooth. Is sugar really that bad for you?

Yes. Sugar is just calories without any good bits added (i. e. vitamins, protein, fibre) and you get the calories that you need with the good bits by eating healthily. We really don't need sugar on its own as this can cause tooth decay. Sugary foods also tend to be high in calories, so eating too much can make you put on weight.

Chemical names for sugar are glucose, sucrose, fructose, dextrose and maltose. None is any better than another nor is brown or cane sugar any better than white.

I've read that poor dental health can cause coronary heart disease – is this true?

Poor dental health is not good for you whichever way you look at the problem. It causes bad breath and can lead to infections. There is a link between poor dental health and coronary heart disease but this may reflect other factors such as poor nutrition, cigarette smoking and generally poor conditions in a person's lifestyle. A recent publication has suggested that even allowing for these other factors, poor dental health can harm the heart. The message is clear – look after your teeth and gums!

Have you any tips for cutting down on sugar?

Cutting down on sugar is the easiest way to begin losing weight whereas cutting down on your fat intake is the most effective (see section below on *Losing weight*).

- Begin by cutting out sugar in tea and coffee. It may be tough at first but after four or five days you will wonder why you ever added sugar. Try to do without artificial sweeteners if you can, or use them only sparingly; some contain sodium (salt) which can upset your blood pressure control or treatment of heart failure.

- Drink low calorie drinks such as Diet Coke or caffeine-free diet coke, Diet 7-Up, diet tonic. Remember plain water is the most refreshing calorie-free drink there is.

- Choose tinned fruit in natural juice rather than syrup.

- Beware of sugar-coated breakfast cereals. A good breakfast could consist of low fat, low calorie yoghurt poured on unsweetened muesli, bran-type cereals with some fresh fruit or porridge made with skimmed or semi-skimmed milk.

- Chocolate, cakes, biscuits and puddings can be replaced by fresh fruit, such as apples, bananas and pears, or low fat yoghurts, fromage frais, low fat mousses and frozen desserts.

Salt

I have raised blood pressure and my doctor tells me that I must cut down on my salt. Why is this?

Excess salt can raise the blood pressure (see Chapter 2). Salt (sodium chloride is the chemical name) in excess causes your body to retain water, upsetting the hormone balance, and the blood pressure goes up.

It is best to avoid extra salt at the table and any salty foods, such as crisps and salted nuts. Table 9.4 gives a guide to salty foods.

Table 9.4 Levels of sodium in various foods

Foods	Typical portion size (g)	Sodium (mg)
Processed foods		
Bacon (grilled)	45	900
Baked beans	200	1060
Bread (2 slices)	75	390
Butter (salted, spread on large slice of bread)	7	61
Cereals		
All-Bran + milk	25 + 115	468
Cornflakes + milk	30 + 115	340
Cheddar cheese	30	183
Corned beef (2 slices)	60	570
Cream cracker + processed cheese	21 + 20	392
Ice-cream	75	54
Mars Bar	65	98
Pork pie (medium)	140	1104
Sausages (2 grilled)	90	900
Sausage roll		332
Scone	50	385
Spaghetti hoops	125	525
Tomato sauce (1 tbsp)	17	58
Tomato soup (canned)	240	1108
Unprocessed foods		
Apples (1 medium dessert, peeled)	120	2
Bananas (1 medium peeled)	100	1
Beef (roast topside, 3 slices)	90	43
Cabbage (boiled, white)	100	4
Carrots		
(boiled, old)	70	35
(tinned)	65	240
Chicken (meat only)	100	81
Cod in batter (fried)	85	85
Eggs (2, scrambled with milk/butter/salt)	140	1442
Potatoes (boiled, old)	150	5
(mashed with butter)	170	83

Table 9.4 Levels of sodium in various foods (*continued*)

Foods	Typical portion size (g)	Sodium (mg)
Drinks		
Beer (1 pint draught bitter)	568 ml	68
Bovril (heaped tsp)	5	240
Coffee (instant)	195	1
Horlicks + semi-skimmed milk	20 + 195	199
Marmite (heaped tsp)	5	225
Milk (2 tbsp)	30	15
Tea (1 cup)	195	Trace

So how much salt do we actually need in our diet?

Your body needs 500 mg of sodium a day, the same as one-third of a teaspoon of salt. We eat on average one to three teaspoons of salt a day equivalent to 6–18 g salt. In the UK, men eat just over 3 g sodium a day, equivalent to six to seven times more than they need.

I know that I eat too much salt and my blood pressure is on the high side. What foods should I try and limit?

When you read a food label, look at the sodium level not just the phrase 'low in salt' (see the questions on food labelling below). See the difference in processed foods which are high in sodium because salt is added during their manufacture (see Table 9.4). Salt gives us sodium – 1 g table salt contains 390 mg sodium. Now compare these with unprocessed foods which are low in sodium but high in potassium. Potassium is helpful in lowering blood pressure. Restriction of both sodium and potassium intake may be advised if you have kidney disease but healthy people usually get rid of any excess. However, if you eat a lot of sodium, this can lead to high blood pressure and fluid retention, which puts a strain on your heart.

Remember, there may be unexpected sources of salt –

monosodium glutamate is often overlooked. Try herbs and spices rather than salt with your cooking. Watch out for:

- snacks, e. g. salted nuts or crisps
- frozen or canned fish (even tuna in brine)
- meat, especially ham or bacon, sausages, corned beef
- canned foods and packet soups
- commercial pies
- some cheeses
- salad dressings.

I have heard that bananas are very good for you. Why is this?

It is true to say that most people are not deficient in either sodium or potassium and a good healthy diet contains more potassium than most of us need. However, potassium-rich foods can help to lower blood pressure and may reduce the need for tablets in some people with high blood pressure. Many fruits like apples, pineapple, grapefruit and raw tomatoes contain potassium; dried raisins and bananas are particularly good sources. Leaf vegetables (spinach, broccoli, brussels sprouts, cabbage, celery and lettuce) are also good sources as are potatoes, parsnips, broad and baked beans. A high intake of potassium is not usually harmful because your kidneys get rid of any excess but, if you have kidney disease or are taking potassium-containing tablets, potassium levels can build up and cause irregular heart beats. Check with your doctor if you are unsure.

Food labels and how to read them

There seems to be a lack of leadership and motivation as regards food labelling – some labels are good, some hardly exist. It is always a problem when healthcare and politics get mixed up.

How do I read food labels and what do the figures mean for me?

It is important to know about salt, fat and calories. Most of the salt that you eat is that added in food manufacturing, so simply watching the salt you add is not enough. Some food labels may specify the sodium content, but it would be impracticable (and difficult) for you to have to add up the sodium content of all manufactured foods that you buy. As a general guide, cut down on salt added in cooking, avoid it at the table and avoid the very salty foods listed above.

Try to keep your daily cholesterol below 300 mg and sodium below 3000 mg(3 g). This is a higher sodium intake than we need but the body copes with this and it is a more practical approach to food. Sodium in grams × 2.5 equals salt in grams; so, 3 g of sodium = 7.5 g of salt and 2.4 g of sodium = 6 g salt. We need 500 mg of sodium a day (500 mg = 0.5 g) and that equals 1.25 g salt or one-third of a teaspoon.

As a reminder, your fat intake varies with calorie advice but for a typical female, who needs 2000 kcal a day, this will be about 70 g of fat, and for a male needing 2500 kcal a day, 95 g of fat. Of these figures, saturated fat should be no more than a third. Table 9.5 is adapted from the American Heart Association Guidelines.

Table 9.5 Guidelines for food intake for average-sized men and women per day

Intake	Men	Women
Energy	2500 kcal	2000 kcal
Total fat*	95 tg	70 g
Saturated fat[†]	30 g	20 g
Fibre	20 tg	16 g
Salt[‡]	6.0 g	5.5 g

* Total fat is 35% of energy.
[†] Total saturated fat is 11% of energy.
[‡] 6.0 g salt equals 2 level teaspoons and 2.4 g sodium.

Table 9.6 Guide to food-type content in 100 g-portions

Food type	A lot (g)	A little (g)
Sugar	10	2
Fat	20	3
Saturated fats	5	1
Fibre	3	0.5
Sodium	0.5	0.1

Here are some guidelines for reading labels.

- Compare figures per 100 g and per serving if you eat the whole pack. You can usually compare product to product per 100 g.

- For each 100 g portion, a simple guide to content is shown in Table 9.6.

- Energy is measured in calories (kilocalories shortened to kcal) and joules (kilojoules shortened to kJ): 1 kcal equals 4.2 kJ. If you take in more calories than you burn up, you will gain weight. See above for your daily needs.

- Proteins are important for your body's building bricks. We all have more than we need except vegetarians, who need to pay more attention to increasing the protein content of their diet to adequate levels.

- Sugar content should be no more than 70 g daily for men and 50 g for women.

An example of a good food label, giving us all the essential information, is given in Table 9.7. Look at the fat, fibre, sugar and sodium content and compare with Table 9.6.

Garlic

I have read that garlic is very good for high blood pressure. Is this true?

There is unfortunately no evidence that garlic reduces cholesterol but it may slightly reduce blood pressure – more research is needed.

The best advice is to make garlic part of your diet, providing of course that you like it and it doesn't limit your social life!

Drinks

I drink quite a few cups of coffee a day. Is coffee bad for the heart?

High caffeine levels can cause palpitations (see Chapter 6). Boiled coffee (percolators) can raise cholesterol but instant, filter or expresso do not. There is no real evidence of any harmful effect of coffee on the coronary arteries. So you can drink and enjoy coffee without worrying about it causing a heart attack. Try to avoid percolated coffee because of the cholesterol effect and cut down on all coffee if you have palpitations.

I like to have a drink now and again. How does alcohol affect my heart?

Alcohol in moderation helps the heart, but in excess it can cause strokes, high blood pressure and cirrhosis of the liver. Alcohol therefore can be consumed without undue worry but it needs to be controlled. Alcohol is, unfortunately, high in calories, so it is not helpful if you are trying to lose weight. Binge drinking is very bad for blood pressure – the following day your blood pressure may be very high and this is when strokes occur.

We measure alcohol in terms of units and it is recommended that men have no more than 28 and women 21 units in a week. Ideally men should not drink more than 4 units a day and women

Table 9.7 An example of a good food label for a breakfast cereal

Ingredients

Wheat, malt extract, sugar, salt, niacin, iron, thiamin (B1), riboflavin (B2), folic acid

Nutrition information

	Typical values per 100 g (3.5 oz)	Typical values per 37.5 g serving with 150 ml semiskimmed milk
Energy	339 kcal	191 kcal
	1439 kJ	811 kJ
Protein	11.5 g	9.1 g
Carbohydrates	67.3 g	31.7 g
of which Sugars	4.7 g	9.2 g
Starch	62.6 g	22.5 g
Fat 2.7 g	3.4 g	
of which Saturates	0.7vg	1.8 g
Mono-unsaturates	0.3 g	0.9 g
Polyunsaturates	1.7 g	0.6 g
Fibre	10.9 g	3.9 g
Sodium	0.3 g	0.2 g
Thiamin (B1)	1.2 mg (85% RDA)	0.5 mg (35% RDA)
Riboflavin (B2)	1.4 mg (85% RDA)	0.8 mg (47% RDA)
Niacin	15.3 mg (85% RDA)	5.7 mg 31% RDA)
Folic acid	170 µg (85% RDA)	70.0 µg (35% RDA)
Iron 11.9 mg (85% RDA)	4.4 mg (31% RDA)	

RDA means Recommended Daily Allowance
Per 37.5@tg serving with 150@tml semiskimmed milk = 191 calories and 3.4@g fat

3 units a day. The British Heart Foundation recommends a weekly limit of 21 units for men and 14 for women. When pouring drinks at home no one ever pours a single shot of spirits unless they use an actual measure – it is always a double or even a treble! One unit of alcohol is equal to:

- one 100 cc glass of wine (red or white) (Note that a bottle of wine at 12.5% volume contains six glasses of 125 ml (a typical measure) and this represents 1.6 units per glass.

- a single measure of sherry
- half a pint of normal strength beer
- quarter of a pint of strong beer
- a single measure of a spirit.

Any form of alcohol benefits the heart (not just red wine) but it must be at a regular acceptable intake – you can't save all your units up for Saturday night! See also the question below on calories in alcohol. Some alcohol now has the units on the can or bottle – this is very helpful and more labels should carry this information.

Always make sure alcohol does not interfere with any medication you might be taking. For example, it increases the effect of warfarin and it interacts with sleeping tablets (increasing their effects) and some pain killers (especially co-proxamol/distalgesic) and some antibiotics (e. g. metronidazole). Alcohol can also increase the drowsiness some people experience with antihistamines (e. g. Piriton).

I have heard a lot about the benefits of wine. Is wine better than beer or spirits?

Unfortunately, this has become confusing with reports contradicting each other. All alcohol is beneficial in moderation. Wine has no advantages over beer. Alcohol is not a medicine and should only be taken if enjoyed.

Snacks

Besides fruit can you suggest some healthy snacks?

For nibbles:

- raw vegetables (cucumber, celery, mangetout, baby corn, broccoli or cherry tomatoes)
- dried fruits (apricots, banana, raisins, sultanas)

- yoghurt (low fat types)

- popcorn (no added salt or sugar).

For more substantial snacks:

- fresh vegetable soups (not cream)

- beans on toast

- baked potatoes (fill with cottage cheese, baked beans or salad)

- wholemeal or soft grain white bread sandwiches with healthy fillings, such as tuna and sweetcorn, turkey and salad, a little Brie cheese and fruit.

Drink water, slimline tonic or tea with lemon or lime.

All these suggestions are not only good for a healthy diet, but also a good way towards losing weight (see section below).

Losing weight

It is easy to start cutting down on calories but keeping to your resolutions is tough. Most people with high blood pressure tend to be overweight. **Losing weight should be a gradual process as part of a lifestyle change – avoid dramatic slimming fads.**

I know I have to lose some weight. Have you any general tips?

Most people know what is fattening and what isn't so you can avoid obvious foods (see Table 9.2) but here are a few tips:

- Losing weight is much easier if at the same time you increase your physical exercise. Taking exercise benefits the heart in general (see Chapter 10).

- Avoid snacking. If you nibble a lot, drink plenty of water, and use fruit or starchy foods (such as a roll with low fat spread) as your filler rather than peanuts or crisps. See the list above for healthy snacks.

- Plan your meals and plan how to avoid temptation. If you are visiting friends for a meal let them know what you are trying to achieve and why. Good friends will be pleased that you confided in them – they will probably be constructive and helpful. If you go to a restaurant, look for those which have courses that fit in with your healthy eating plan.

- If you develop a craving (a choc attack!), reach for that apple and go for a walk. Repeat to yourself what you are doing and why.

- If you slip, don't give up, regroup and get back on course.

- Avoid too much alcohol – instead of a gin and tonic have a slimline tonic. Have one glass of wine, not two. (See the question below on alcohol.)

- Eat slowly and take your time over the meal.

- Have a salad (with a low calorie dressing) with the meal.

- Always eat breakfast. Porridge is a good low calorie filler. Use semiskimmed milk. Cereals vary a lot as regards calorie content – read the label carefully rather than the marketing message.

- Don't miss meals or have one big meal a day.

- Don't shop when you are hungry and always take a shopping list with you rather than go for impulse buying.

- Use a smaller plate when serving.

- Stick a photograph of *how you want to be* on the fridge. It will help you to avoid temptation as you visualize the new slimmer you!

- Slim with a friend or join a reputable slimming club – group support can be very motivating

- Eat healthy foods (as discussed in the **Food types and eating healthily** section above).

- Always cut the fat off food and do not cook in fat. Avoid fried foods. (See the advice above on the best ways to cook food.)

- If you do use fat for cooking, use a healthier oil (such as olive oil) which is high in unsaturated fats (see Chapter 2). Shallow-fry in the minimum of oil to get the maximum benefit. Use a non-stick frying pan and do not overheat. If you deep fry, use a 'good' oil and replace the oil after five uses.

- Keep away from cakes, chocolates, biscuits and any pastries or pies.

- Choose plainer biscuits, such as rich tea or marie types.

- Have a fresh fruit salad, fruit tinned in natural juices, fromage frais, low fat mousse or frozen yoghurt for dessert.

How quickly should I lose weight?

Aim for no more than 1 kg (2 lb) a week – a gradual change is more likely to be sustained and it is healthier.

My friend has taken so-called diet tablets. Do these work?

Eating healthily and weight loss are about making lifestyle changes, so drugs should be avoided if at all possible. Some drugs are addictive and others may damage the heart valves. Many that are sold for high prices are capsules of nonsense. Xenical (orlistat), however, has research behind it. It may help obese people as part of a lifestyle change. It goes with a properly controlled low fat diet and works by inhibiting the absorption of 30% of the fat eaten. Side effects include bowel disturbances. Xenical is part of a carefully controlled (supervised by a dietician) diet, and is a course of tablets, not a long-term treatment. It is not a magic slimming bullet, but it does have an important role for a small number of obese people.

I have been on a slimming diet and managed to lose some weight. How can I keep the weight off now?

First of all remember why you lost it – you have lowered your blood pressure and reduced the strain on your heart. So praise yourself. You will feel better and that alone will give you the incentive you need to keep slim and fit.

Other tips include:

- Maintain regular exercise, walking briskly, cycling, swimming (see Chapter 10).

- Keep eating sensibly: plan your meals and follow the plan carefully.

- Eat more starchy foods (e. g. an extra slice or two of bread a day) to prevent you losing more weight if you have reached your target. Do not be tempted to turn to the chocolates again!

- At parties or business lunches, if there is a buffet, choose carefully and don't overeat just because the size of the spread is tempting (and free!) (see question below on eating out).

- If hunger strikes, drink a glass of water and eat fruit – *don't* open the fridge door.

If you start gaining weight, look carefully at what you are eating and how much you exercise – what have you changed? If you lose weight below your target, gradually increase your calorie intake first of all by 200 kcal a day (e. g. an apple is 60 kcal, a slice of bread 80 kcal – there are many 'calorie counting' booklets on the market, listing various foods both raw and packaged); after a week, check it again and keep exercising.

I have seen two different charts for an ideal weight. What should my target weight be?

Your ideal weight must take into account your height (Figure 9.1). Doctors work to your Body Mass Index or BMI. This is your weight in kilograms divided by the square of your height in metres:

$$\text{BMI} = \frac{\text{weight in kg}}{(\text{height in metres})^2} = \frac{\text{kg}}{\text{m}^2}$$

A normal BMI is 20–25. It works well for people over 1.6 m (5 ft 3 in) up to 1.87 m (6 ft 2 in) but not so well for short or tall people. Ask your doctor or his nurse to help you work out your BMI and set your own target BMI. Now check it against your bathroom scales which are not as accurate but which will still show any changes. You can work out what you weigh in kilograms which is equally a guide to your BMI. For example, say that your BMI is 27 and that you want to get to 25, work out your kg at each BMI point and then, using your bathroom scales, all you need to do is set your kg target, as you know what BMI it represents. If you are not sure what to do or how to do it, ask your nurse at the doctor's surgery to help you. Here is an example to help you:

A 1.87 m (6 ft 2 in) man weighs 95 kg. His calculated BMI is:

$$\frac{95}{1.87 \times 1.87} = 27.2$$

He would like to be healthier with a BMI of 24–25 so the calculation is:

$$24 = \frac{?\,\text{kg}}{1.87 \times 1.87} \quad \text{i.e. } 84\,\text{kg}$$

He now knows what to aim for on his scales.

Check your weight once a week only and aim to lose 1 kg (2.2 lb) in the first week and then 0.5 kg a week thereafter. If you use bathroom scales, do not put them on a carpet, and check them against a known weight from time to time (e. g. bags of flour). Compare them with your doctor's scales or a large one in a chemist's shop.

I find the whole business of BMI confusing – can't it be made simpler?

Of course. Simply follow the height and weight chart. Another simple formula is:

- Height in cm minus 110 = optimal weight in kg for men
- Height in cm minus 100 = optimal weight in kg for women.

So, if you are male measuring 5 ft 10 in, convert your height to centimetres (177.8 cm), take away 110 and you reach 67.8 kg. This is your ideal weight.

I have heard the nurse talk about a waist/hip ratio. What is this? Does it apply to my husband as well as me?

If your tummy is fat, the risk of heart problems increases and you can calculate the risk by comparing the waist measurement with that at the hip. You divide your waist measurement by your hip measurement. So, if your waist measures 26 in and hip 34 in, then you would have a ratio of 0.76 (26 divided by 34); you would not be at risk because the safe ratio for women should be no more than 0.8; this means that your waist should not be more than 80% of your hip measurement. Put another way being apple-shaped is bad but pear-shaped is positively good!

The ratio for your husband, say with a 40 in waist and a 34 in hip, is calculated by dividing 40 by 34 which equals 1.18. He would be at risk because the safe ratio for men should be no more than 1.0. So his waist should not be greater than his hip measurement or the ratio would be over 1.0. Having a belly that's bigger than your hips increases your risks of getting coronary artery disease.

For men, if your waist is 37–40 in, you are overweight; over 40 in and you are fat (politely known as obese). In women, if the waist is 32–35 in, you are overweight, and over 35 in, you are fat.

Use the chart or do this calculation to find out your BMI: divide your weight in kilograms by the square of your height in metres.

Your BMI score:
below 20: underweight
20–25: ideal
25–30: overweight
30+: seriously overweight – you need to see your doctor

Figure 9.1 What you should weigh. Take a straight line up from your height (without shoes) and across your weight (without clothes), and put a mark where the lines meet. How did you do?

I've tried all sorts of slimming diets and nothing seems to work – what can I do now?

Trying a slimming diet is not the right way of tackling weight reduction – it is a lifestyle change that is needed. If you cannot do it on your own, don't give up. Join one of the groups such as Weight Watchers and attend regularly. Remember why you need to lose weight: your blood pressure will benefit and you will reduce your chances of a stroke or heart attack.

Is it safe for heart patients to try the Atkins diet?

The Atkins diet is high fat, high protein and low carbohydrate. The theory is that when we eat carbohydrates and sugar the body responds by making insulin to burn them off. Too much intake equals too much insulin and then too much fat is stored and therefore we gain weight. In the short term it works for many people but there is a tendency towards constipation and bad breath. Heart patients with high cholesterol levels are usually protected by statins but control can be lost. My view is that if there is significant weight loss, this is good in the short term – say 2–3 months – but for long-term protection a switch should be made to the Mediterranean Diet, which is proven to cut the risks of a heart attack and is the programme described in this chapter.

We have a local WeightWatchers group in our area. Are slimming groups any good?

Any group like this can be helpful because of the supportive role and the sensible advice they offer. They reinforce some basic rules.

- Eat less fat and sugar.
- Avoid nibbles.
- Do not miss meals.
- Eat more fruit and vegetables.

- Fill up on low fat high fibre foods.

- Take regular dynamic exercise such as walking, cycling, swimming – any strong movement exercise.

You have mentioned before that Asians have a higher incidence of coronary disease and diabetes – what dietary changes can they make?

It is true that Asians in particular are vulnerable to coronary disease and diabetes. They often have abdominal obesity. Try these tips:

- Fried foods should be avoided.

- Eat low fat yoghurt, semiskimmed or skimmed milk and reduced fat cheeses instead of full fat versions.

- Try casseroling, boiling, grilling, steaming, poaching or microwave cooking instead of adding fat or oil. Some vegetables soak up more oil in during cooking, e.g. fenugreek (methi), aubergines and karelas.

- Try to make minced meat dishes and dhals without fat and avoid using oil in the cooking.

- Remove visible fat from meats.

- Do not spread fat on chapattis and do not add oil or ghee to the chapatti dough. Reduce Indian deep fried snacks such as chevdon, sev, samosas, puris, pakoras and chips.

- Switch from creamy salad dressing to low-fat yoghurt based dressing.

There is an excellent information sheet on this website: www.heartuk.org.uk (number 03).

We have a full social life and I am often out during the week at business lunches. How can I avoid fatty foods when I am out?

If you are going to family or friends, tell your host that you have been told to lose weight and what you need to do about it. They will understand and because they now will know that you don't eat fatty foods or sweet desserts, any embarrassment will be avoided.

At a restaurant:

- Avoid the cocktails (tomato juice and mineral water are just as fashionable these days).

- Avoid fried appetizers or cream soups – select minestrone or gazpacho soups.

- Choose a fresh fruit starter such as melon.

- Look for the grilled fish or poultry and ask for any sauces to be left off.

- Grilled Dover sole and a salad are a good standby.

- Remove the skin from poultry and don't eat fatty meat.

- Take a salad with vinegar and oil instead of mayonnaise.

- At a salad bar, avoid cream dressings, cheese, olives, bacon bits and croûtons.

- Have fresh vegetables such as spinach or carrots. Ask for sauces or butter to be left off vegetables or put 'on the side'.

- Order baked or boiled new potatoes in their skins.

- At Oriental restaurants, have a stir-fry of chicken or fish and vegetables. Steamed rice is better than fried. Resist sweet 'n sour dishes and banana/apple fritters.

- In Italian restaurants, avoid creamy sauces.

- In Indian restaurants, have plain tandoori or tikka with a salad and steamed or boiled rice, rather than those dishes

which come in thick sauces. Indian cooking involves a lot
of fat and sometimes coconut so, in general, menu options
should be very carefully selected. Ask if you are not sure
how certain dishes are cooked.

- Dessert can be fresh fruit or sorbet – try to avoid cream.

- Enjoy a glass of wine and perhaps finish with black coffee
  (decaffeinated if you are prone to palpitations – see
  Chapter 6).

Some restaurants now have items marked as being low in fat.
Airlines also often offer this when meal options are presented.

If you are the host, you can choose the restaurant. If you are a
regular at a particular restaurant, tell the owner about your
preferences so that you will be able to eat without drawing
attention to any question mark over your health.

There are times when I really fancy a steak. Should I never eat this?

An occasional treat is fine. Make sure it is a grilled fillet with the
fat removed. If you are not sure what to eat, always go for the
healthy option but, if after a while you feel you 'could murder a
steak', enjoy one, but don't overdo it. Remember, a 170–225 g
(6–8 oz) fillet steak is the best weight to go for.

What should my intake of fats be?

Your saturated fat intake should represent no more than 10% of
your total calories; polyunsaturated fats should make up 10% and
monounsaturated fats 10–15%. As 1 g of fat equals 9 kcal:

- if your daily calorie intake is 1500 kcal, you need only 50 g
  of fat at most;

- if it is 2000 kcal you need 65–70 g of fat, and

- if it is 2500 kcal, you need 85–90 g of fat.

Can you give some simple guidelines regarding calories? How many should I need on a daily basis?

To calculate the number of calories to maintain your weight now, multiply the number of pounds you weigh by 13 kcal if you don't take much exercise, and by 15 if you do. The equivalent figures if you calculate in kilograms are 29 and 33 respectively.

To lose 1 lb you need to burn up 3500 kcal (1 kg = 7700) and this means reducing your daily intake by 500 kcal to lose 1 lb in one week (0.5 kg = 550). You can cut down 500 kcal by, for example, cutting out a can of coke, a chocolate bar or 4 teaspoons of sugar.

Weigh yourself once a week and adjust your intake accordingly. Always combine weight loss with a healthy increase in physical activity. For example, if you walk briskly at 4 miles per hour for 2 miles, you will use up 300 kcal.

If you fall below your target weight, increase your calorie intake by 200 kcal a day (around a couple of slices of bread and a thin slice of lean ham) but keep up the exercise programme.

I know I should eat more vegetables and fruit in my diet to lose weight. Which ones have the least calories?

Nearly all vegetables and fruits in general are low in calories and high in nutrients and vitamins. Vegetables are encouraged because they are very nutritious and low in calories, so you can really go to town with them! They are packed with protein and great for using instead of meat dishes (e. g. lentil lasagne) or to pad out meat-based meals (e. g. chilli con carne). You do not really need to count the calories but, as a guide, an average portion of the following vegetables is equal to about 20 kcal:

Asparagus	Mushrooms
Aubergine	Onions
Green beans	Parsnips
Broccoli	Peas
Brussels sprouts	Peppers
Cabbage	Radishes
Carrots	Spinach

Cauliflower
Celery
Cucumber/courgette
Lettuce

Tomatoes
Turnips
Vegetable juices

The following fruits are each equal to 60 kcal:

1 apple
4 apricots
1 banana
12 cherries
2 plums
3 prunes
2 tangerines
2 tablespoons of raisins

1 nectarine
1 orange
1 peach
3 dates
2 figs
½ grapefruit
15 grapes
½ mango

1 portion blackberries/melon/pineapple/strawberries/raspberries

If you buy tinned fruit, make sure that they are in natural juices, not syrup.

What exactly is a 'portion'?

A portion is one large fruit (such as an apple, orange or banana); two small fruits (such as plums or satsumas); 1 cup of raspberries, strawberries or grapes; 1 glass (150 ml) of fruit juice; 1 tbsp of dried fruit; 2 tbsp of raw cooked or frozen vegetables or 1 dessert bowl of salad.

I know there is a good deal of fibre in breads and cereals. What about their calorie value?

The following are equal to 80 kcal:

- 1 slice of bread
- 1 portion of bran cereal (e. g. All-Bran, one Shredded Wheat) without milk
- 1 portion of pasta or rice.

Remember that high fibre starchy foods are valuable parts of a healthy lifestyle as we have already discussed.

How many calories are there in alcohol?

A glass of wine is 100 kcal, a pint of beer 400 and a single measure of spirit 100, whereas slimline tonic is at most 1 calorie and water contains nil. Unsweetened fresh fruit juice and sparkling water are very good alternatives to alcohol when you are trying to watch your weight.

I want to be healthy and not overweight – can you summarize for me the most important ways of achieving this?

It is important to think of any change as a healthy change to your lifestyle. Losing weight must be a part of a change to healthy food and a regular exercise programme. It is really a healthy way of living rather than just losing weight. To achieve this, here are the basic rules:

- Eat lots of fruit and vegetables every day.
- High fibre foods are filling, healthy and low in fat.
- Try to avoid fatty foods, such as bacon, sausages and pies.
- When you have poultry, do not eat the skin.
- Avoid cakes and crisps, which contain a lot of fat.
- Use low fat yoghurt or fromage frais instead of cream.
- When you cook, steam, grill, bake or microwave food instead of frying.
- When you have canned fish, drain off the oil (your cat would like this!) or use those that come in brine.
- When you have pasta, use tomato-based vegetable sauce rather than creamy sauces.
- When you use fats, even polyunsaturated or olive oil, use it sparingly.
- Try not to nibble nuts.

- Eat slowly.

- Use a smaller plate.

- Cut down on alcohol; drink plenty of water.

- Don't replace meals by snacks – always eat breakfast.

- Don't shop when you are hungry.

- Don't be depressed if you slip up – regroup and start again the next day.

- Try to take dynamic exercise three times a week for at least 30 minutes.

If I miss a meal because I am travelling or I am on business, what can you suggest as an alternative?

Cereal bars, fig rolls, nuts, oat biscuits and rice cakes provide low-fat energy. Fruit is always a good standby – an apple a day may well keep the doctor away after all!

10
Exercise

Why bother?

Most people get little vigorous exercise either at work or during
their leisure time. We travel by car, bus or train, and at the end of
the day we flop down in front of the TV. There is now a lot of
evidence that regular exercise of low or moderate intensity, done
on a regular basis (daily if possible, four to five times a week
otherwise), can reduce the risk of getting heart disease. Activities
that benefit the heart include walking, climbing stairs, gardening,

264

housework such as making the beds or vacuuming the stairs not just wafting a feather duster, dancing or using home or gym exercise equipment. Increasing your exercise to be more vigorous helps further improve your heart and lungs – brisk walking, cycling, swimming, skipping or running (jogging) are easy examples that can become part of your everyday lifestyle.

Throughout this book the importance of exercise for the heart has been stressed. It really does help to be fit. If you find it a struggle to exercise on your own, get the whole family to join in and be supportive. Otherwise:

- Join a sports or leisure club.
- Do any exercise that you enjoy.
- Try a new sport such as golf.
- Clean your car yourself, not in a car wash.
- Get working in the garden if you have one – 30 minutes in the fresh air digging or weeding in the fresh air is excellent exercise.
- Swim with a friend or relative.
- Get the bicycle out of storage – have it serviced if necessary, and buy the right safety kit before trying it out on a quiet road at first if you don't feel confident.
- If you have an exercise bicycle, stop hanging clothes on it and start using it.
- Don't give up – every little helps.
- Keep working at it.
- Always be positive.

Remember that exercise should be enjoyed, not endured. You should be able to find some form of exercise that you really enjoy.

Why will exercise do me good?

There are many reasons why exercise is so good for everyone:

- It will help you lose and maintain your optimal weight.

- It increases your good cholesterol (HDL).

- It helps smokers stop smoking.

- It lowers blood pressure and thus helps prevent heart disease.

Physically fit people are usually psychologically fit also. Fit people feel better, live longer and have less heart disease. They also sleep better and handle stress better.

What types of exercise are good for the heart? I have been doing weight lifting for years – is it of any help to my heart?

Activities that involve movement are known as dynamic or aerobic exercise and these are the ones that benefit the heart (walking, cycling, swimming etc.). Aerobic means that the body uses oxygen to deliver the energy that you need for the activity that you are performing. Aerobic exercise for at least 30 minutes four or five times a week will strengthen your heart and help to reduce your chance of developing coronary artery disease.

Weight lifting is a form of static exercise, also known as isometric or akinetic exercise. This does not help the heart and can put on unnatural strain on it by raising your blood pressure. Other examples of static exercise are pushing a car that won't start, lifting heavy bags without help, moving furniture on your own – you know that with a big effort you can do it, but if you wait for help there will less strain on your heart.

Building up your muscles without dynamic exercise may make the outside of your chest look good but it will not help the heart inside. Those ill-advised people who take steroids can actually damage their hearts because steroids sometimes weaken the heart muscle so that it becomes flabby. Anabolic steroids can cause the blood to clot more easily and a heart attack becomes more likely.

I've read about exercise and there is often a mention of METs – what are they?

A MET is short for 'metabolic equivalent'. This is a measure of the work the body does when exercising – the more you work at exercise, the more METs you use. Sitting watching the TV equals 1 MET, walking will use up to 5 METs depending on how brisk it is, and running will use even more (Table 10.1). When we exercise we achieve our personal limit depending on how fit we are, and this is known as our 'functional capacity'. As our fitness improves, so does our functional capacity.

If I'm fit why should I quit smoking as well?

No risk factor works on its own. Getting fit goes along with losing weight, not smoking, avoiding fatty foods and moderating alcohol. If you smoke you are three times more likely to get coronary artery disease. Smoking is a bigger cause of heart disease than lack of exercise. So if you are super fit but smoke 10–20 cigarettes a day, the smoking will win the argument and you will lose out – being fit does not allow you to smoke.

I am now 51 and made a resolution on my 50th birthday to take exercise regularly. I found that my good intentions fell away after 3 months when I was ill for a week with 'flu. What do you suggest might help now?

First of all it is important not to exercise when you are ill, so you did the right thing when you had 'flu. Start again with a practice walk for about a mile, going slowly, then try and reduce the time that this length takes. Keep a record. If you walk on a footpath by a roadway, you can measure the distance using a car; if you walk in the countryside, select a path where the distance is shown.

If you walk for 1 mile at 2 mph, you will take 30 minutes and use up 2.5 METs, which isn't much effort but it is an important beginning. At 3 mph it will take you 20 minutes and use 3.5 METs; at 4 mph it will take 15 minutes and use 4.5 METs. When you are walking fast and just out of breath, fitness will be achieved for the

Table 10.1 Activities and their metabolic equivalents

Activity	METs
Aerobics	
low impact	5
high impact	7
Badminton	4.5
Bowling	4
Cycling	
< 10 mph	4
10–12 mph	6
> 12 mph	10
DIY (e.g. wallpapering)	4–5
Football	8
Gardening (e.g. digging)	3–5
Golf	4–5
Horse riding (trotting)	5–7
Housework (average)	2.5
scrubbing floors	5.5
Playing the piano	2.5
Office job	1.5
Sex ('normal')	2–3
Sex ('vigorous')	3–6
Skiing	
downhill racing	8
leisure	6
Squash	12
Swimming	
fast	10
moderate	8
light	6
butterfly	11
Table tennis	4
Tennis	8
Walking (1 mile in 20 min)	3

over-40s at about 5 METs for men and women – this is equivalent to walking 2 miles in 30 minutes.

I'm over 60 and have never really taken exercise properly, though I live an outdoor life. Am I too old to exercise now?

Age should not be a limitation to anybody starting to take exercise although it is better to have exercised throughout your life. Exercise will keep you feeling and looking younger longer. If you haven't exercised before or are starting again after a long gap, just remember to build up gradually. Always check with your doctor first, if you are at all uncertain as to whether a particular form of exercise is suitable for you.

I am going to start an exercise routine. How will I be able to work out how many calories I use up?

This depends on the type of exercise you take and for how long:

- If you walk at 3 miles an hour (about normal walking speed), you will burn up 320 kcal per hour.

- If you walk at 4.5 mph (pretty fast, almost a jog), this goes up to 440 kcal per hour.

- If you cycle at 6 mph, you will burn 240 kcal per hour.

- If you swim 25 yards (a length of most swimming pools) in a minute, you will burn 275 kcal per hour.

The fatter you are, the more you burn, and you burn more if you exercise for longer rather than faster (e. g. cycling at 12 mph burns 410 kcal per hour not 480).

How much?

I have a busy life and am not sure that I can set aside half an hour every day for exercising. Is my effort wasted if I do not take exercise every day?

You must begin slowly – you cannot become an athlete overnight – and increase gradually. The aim is to perform any aerobic exercise for 30–40 minutes four to five times a week. Even relatively modest exercise is good, such as gardening, housework and dancing, but it is better if you can develop a walking programme to include both distance and speed as well as enjoyment (see below for a good programme to follow).

Try to exercise at least every other day and more at the weekend (a walk in the country at the weekend will be fun and less polluted than a city walk). Try to make it a regular commitment, e. g. in your lunch hour, especially if your workplace offers showers. Afterwards, have a glass of water. Ask a friend or partner to join in. Keep a record to judge your progress. Dancing can be quite vigorous (e. g. country dancing), so it is a particularly good form of exercise because you can build up from gentler beginnings. It is also exercise with a good social side to it.

I am put off exercising because, in my exercise class, everyone else seems much fitter than me. Why is this?

Life is like that! Everyone at first seems fitter! They may have been working at it longer. You are the most important person and you should focus purely on your own programme. Don't worry what everybody else is doing. It is not a competition. Don't be embarrassed, get stuck in. They were probably unfit once and so they will be supportive.

Safety

You mention talking to my doctor before I start exercising. Do I really need a medical check first?

If you have no medical problems, the answer is no – get out and start straight away. If you've already had heart trouble or don't know about your blood pressure, get this checked by your doctor and ask for a cholesterol check while you are there. If you are 'at risk' (e. g. over 60 years, a smoker, have diabetes or on medication for your heart), it's best to check with your doctor first.

I'm worried that I might overdo things. Should I take any special precautions before exercising?

- Don't exercise if you feel unwell, e. g. if you've had 'flu or a bad cold. If you have had any recent illness, go back to exercising only when you have recovered and then build up slowly.

- If you get chest pain or breathing trouble while you are exercising, see your doctor.

- Don't exercise after a heavy meal or a hot bath – wait two to three hours before doing any.

- Avoid caffeine and alcohol for an hour before and after exercise.

Last time I tried jogging, I tore a calf muscle and was off work for 2 weeks. How can I avoid this happening again?

Don't exercise too hard too quickly and always loosen up first (see the warm-up exercises below) and do some cooling down exercises last (walk slowly for 3–5 minutes, stretch for 2 minutes). Never overdo it. One of the best things to do is to buy the correct shoes for the sport you are choosing (see question later regarding special clothing for exercising).

Choosing your exercise

My local recreation centre offers 40 different sports from judo to meditation. What is the best form of exercise to do?

Any aerobic exercise is the best. This is dynamic exercise using large groups of muscles – for example walking, jogging, cycling and swimming. Non-aerobic exercise builds muscle strength (what is known as *isometrics*) but does little to help the heart's fitness and can be harmful, as it can make your blood pressure rise.

I lead a very busy life and just do not have time to exercise. Is there anything I can do?

Your health should always come first. No one on his death bed wished he'd spent more time at the office! However, you can exercise around your work commitments.

- Climb the stairs rather than take the lift.
- Park so that you have to walk 200–300 yards to work.
- If you use public transport, get off the bus, train or tube a stop early and walk to or from the station.

I am in my forties and have always hated competitive sport but enjoy walking. Is there a simple walking programme I could start?

Walking is especially good because it is cheap and generally safe and we all know how to do it. It also doesn't strain the joints as much as jogging or running. The American Heart Association walking programme (Table 10.2) is useful (but not compulsory), so you can vary the timing to your personal needs. 'Health Walks' are being developed by the Countryside Commission and the British Heart Foundation (see Appendix 2 for addresses).

(a) Shoulder: shrug – circle (b) Neck: turn – tilt

(c) Spine: bend – turn   (d) Knee: lift   (e) Ankle: heel – toe

Figure 10.1 Warm-up exercises.

You will need a yardstick to assess your progress. Try to find a distance of about one mile (cancel the newspaper and go each day to collect it) – the distance you can measure by car or by striding out and counting the yards or metres. Alternatively, estimate the distance to the park, round the park or to the shops or station.

- Gently loosen up by bending and stretching (Figure 10.1). Repeat exercises 1–5 up to six times before you start walking.

Table 10.2 A simple walking programme

Weeks	Warm-up walking	Target zone walking*
Week 1		
Session A	5 min	briskly, 5 min
Session B	Repeat above pattern	
Session C	Repeat above pattern	

Continue with at least three exercise sessions during each week of the programme.

Week 2	5 min	briskly, 7 min
Week 3	5 min	briskly, 9 min
Week 4	5 min	briskly, 11 min
Week 5	5 min	briskly, 13 min
Week 6	5 min	briskly, 15 min
Week 7	5 min	briskly, 18 min
Week 8	5 min	briskly, 20 min
Week 9	5 min	briskly, 23 min
Week 10	5 min	briskly, 26 min
Week 11	5 min	briskly, 28 min
Week 12	5 min	briskly, 30 min

Week 13 on:
Check your pulse periodically to see if you are exercising within your target zone. As you become more fit, try exercising within the upper range of your target zone. Gradually increase your brisk walking time to 30–60 min, three or four times a week, Remember that your goal is to get the benefits that you are seeking and enjoy your activity.

*Your target zone is shown in Table 10.3.

- Measure your heart rate by taking your pulse at the wrist or next to your Adam's apple. Count the number in 15 seconds and multiply by 4 or count the number in 6 seconds and add a 0. You now have the beats per minute (Figure 10.2).

- After walking for 5 minutes take your pulse again and speed up to get it above 110. If you are on a beta-blocker drug, this does not apply as these drugs slow the heart. Try to keep the pulse over 110 and note the time you took to

Cool down walking	Total time
more slowly, 5 min	15 min
5 min	17 min
5 min	19 min
5 min	21 min
5 min	23 min
5 min	25 min
5 min	28 min
5 min	30 min
5 min	33 min
5 min	36 min
5 min	38 min
5 min	40 min

complete your mile; take your pulse again whilst winding down. It should settle within 10 minutes.

- As you get fit your walking time should shorten and your heart rate become slower and your recovery become quicker. You can then extend up to two miles, gradually increasing your walking speed and then your distance. Do not do too much too quickly.

Figure 10.2 Taking your pulse at your wrist **(a)** and neck **(b)**.

A friend of mine was told to judge his exercise by the talking test. What is this?

This is a simple but useful guide to how much exercise you are doing. You should be exercising in such a way that you can talk, but you should be a little breathless. If you can talk easily, you are not exercising briskly enough; if you cannot talk, you need to slow down.

I should like to go walking but I'm afraid to walk alone – I'm always reading in the local paper of women being attacked. Isn't it rather dangerous to walk on my own?

It is a sad reflection on the world that people, particularly women, should be afraid to go walking. Attacks do occur but are rare. We always need to keep a sense of proportion – only the bad things get reported. If, of 10 000 women walking in the countryside, only one was attacked, 9999 did not, but we would only hear of the one who suffered. Being afraid is understandable, but in the end it ruins *your* enjoyment of life. If you are worried, why not walk with two or three friends, or join a rambling club. Other precautions could include:

- Carry an alarm or a mobile phone.

- Do not go out when it's getting dark – pick the clear daylight hours.

- Avoid remote areas and keep to open spaces (e. g. the paths in the park).

- Choose the areas where there are lots of people (e. g. along a sea front or a popular park).

I've tried walking 1 mile a day and I find that I get bored after a month. What else can I do besides walking?

Joining a gym will give you access to a treadmill which will give you a better chance to judge your progress more accurately because of its computerized timing.

Other good exercises include rowing, swimming, cycling, dancing (aerobics) or simply climbing stairs. Variety is the thing!

There is a heart testing machine at my local gym, but frankly I do not understand what the figures mean. What should my maximum heart rate be?

Your maximum heart rate should be 220 minus your age. You should aim to get up to 75% of this. So, if you are aged 50, you should aim for three quarters of 170, i. e. 127. When you begin your exercise programme, aim for 50% in the first 6–8 weeks and gradually build up to the 75%. Your target heart rate varies with age (Table 10.3).

This guide applies to healthy people – those aiming to prevent heart disease. Those with heart disease should follow medical advice and limit activity based on awareness of breathing while still comfortable. Beta-blockers slow the heart rate for example, so using the pulse will not be a good guide. Most people with heart problems can ignore the heart rate and exercise with the aim of progressively increasing performance.

Table 10.3 Target heart rates

Age (years)	Target heart rate (bpm*)
20	100–150
30	95–142
40	90–135
50	85–127
60	80–120
70	75–113

*bpm: beats per minute

I've got a tracksuit and trainers. Do I need any other special clothing to exercise in?

If you are going to build up a walking programme, you will need good shoes – don't cut corners in footwear. Walking or jogging shoes are the best, or proper walking boots if you are walking in the countryside. Wear thick socks when you try them on and look for shoes with cushion soles and an arch support. In warm weather, wear cool lightweight cotton and remember to put sunscreen skin cream on to guard against sunburn. In cooler weather, wear two or three layers (a vest, a T-shirt and a sweat-shirt, for example) to retain the heat. Loose-fitting tracksuit bottoms are comfortable and inexpensive. Don't feel you have to go out in the rain – the exercise is to be enjoyed not endured.

Does regular exercise help prevent me from getting a heart attack during sex?

This is another good reason to get fit – physically fit people are sexually fit too and have far less risk of a heart problem during sex. Do you need another excuse?!

What is exercise 'with a purpose'?

Some people need a reason for everything and can't see the point of just taking exercise – they get bored and lose interest. Exercise with a purpose gives them a reason, for example walking to the newsagent for the daily paper, walking the dog, cleaning the car, getting off public transport early and walking the rest of the way to work and playing a sport such as tennis. All exercise like this is good for you. Remember alcohol in moderation is good for you, so walking as briskly as possible to and from the wine shop is exercise with a very good purpose!

Glossary

Aneurysm Sac-like ballooning out of an artery wall, or scar tissue in the heart muscle.

Angina Chest pain when the heart fails to get sufficient blood. Pain is usually a choking sensation which may spread to the jaw or arms.

Angiography X-ray examination of the heart and coronary arteries. Under local anaesthetic, a catheter (fine tube) is passed to the heart and a dye shows up any narrowings or weaknesses. Also known as 'cardiac catheterization'.

Angioplasty Method of removing narrowings in arteries by the temporary insertion of a catheter with a tiny balloon on it. The balloon is inflated to squash the narrowing out of the way.

Angiotensin converting enzyme (ACE inhibitor) Drug that lowers blood pressure and improves heart failure symptoms as well as life expectancy.

Anticoagulant Drug that thins the blood (e. g. warfarin, heparin) and reduces its capacity to clot.

Antioxidant Substance (e. g. vitamin C and E) which prevents fats becoming oxidized and thus allows the fats to build up on the arteries.

Aorta Main artery which leaves the heart and runs down the back of the heart to the abdomen.

Aortic valve Valve between the muscle pump on the left side of the heart (left ventricle) and the aorta.

Arrhythmia Abnormal heart beat.

Artery Vessel carrying oxygen rich blood under pressure. Arterioles are small arteries.

Atheroma (atherosclerosis) Fatty deposits on the lining of blood vessels (plaque).

Atria Two upper chambers of the heart: left atrium and right atrium.

Atrial fibrillation Chaotic heart beats arising in the atria. Always irregular.

Atrial septal defect Hole in the heart between the right and left atria.

Atrioventricular node Junction box in the electrical system of the heart, which helps prevent rapid heart beats affecting the pump's action by limiting the number of beats that can get through.

Automatic implantable cardioverter defibrillator *see* Defibrillator

Beta-blockers Drugs that block adrenaline thereby slowing the heart rate and lowering blood pressure. Used to treat angina, raised blood pressure, heart attacks and palpitations.

Biopsy Removing a tissue sample.

Blood clot Process where blood cells stick together like a jelly (or form a scab on the skin). It protects us from blood loss, but in the wrong place causes heart attacks.

Blood pressure Pressure of the blood in the arteries.

Blood vessels Tubes (arteries or veins) through which blood flows.

Brachial artery Artery at the elbow used for blood pressure measurement.

Bradycardia Slow heart rate (less than 60 beats per minute).

Bundle branch block When one of the electric bundles in the heart is interrupted. There are two bundles, a right and left, and the block is described as right or left bundle branch block – abbreviated to RBBB or LBBB.

Calcium antagonist (or blocker) Drugs that relax arteries by reducing calcium in the walls. Some also reduce irregular heart beats. All lower blood pressure and help angina.

Capillaries Smallest blood vessels joining arteries to veins.

Cardiac Relating to the heart.

Cardiac arrest A heart attack – when the heart suddenly stops beating and pumping blood.

Cardiac catheter Fine tube threaded through an artery to the heart.

Cardiac enzymes Enzymes looked for in a blood test to check for a heart attack.

Cardiac output Amount of blood pumped by the heart each minute. Usually 5 litres.

Cardiology Study of the heart in health and disease.

Cardiologist Doctor specializing in heart disease – a physician not a surgeon.

Cardiomyopathy Disease which weakens heart muscle.

Cardiopulmonary bypass When a machine takes over the heart's work of pumping during surgery.

Cardiovascular Relating to the heart and its blood vessels.

Cardioversion Electric shock treatment for the heart, attempting to convert irregular rhythm to normal.

Carotid arteries Main arteries running up both sides of the neck to the brain.

Cerebral embolism Blood clot which has travelled to the brain.

Cerebral haemorrhage Bleeding into the brain from a ruptured blood vessel.

Cerebral thrombosis Blood clot blocking an artery to the brain.

Cerebrovascular accident Death of brain tissue from a clot or a bleed.

Cholesterol Fatty substance needed for cell building. Too much causes narrowed arteries. *See also* High density lipoprotein; Low density lipoprotein.

Claudication Pain in the legs while walking caused by a lack of oxygen mainly from narrowed arteries – 'angina of the legs'.

Collateral circulation ('collaterals') New small arteries which develop to bypass blocked ones.

Conduction system Electrics of the heart.

Congenital defects Heart problems (structural) that one is born with.

Congestive heart failure *see* Heart failure

Coronary arteries Arteries supplying blood to the heart.

Coronary artery bypass graft (CABG) Surgery using vein or arteries to bypass narrowings or blockages in the coronary arteries.

Coronary artery disease (CAD) Narrowing of the coronary arteries from fatty deposits.

Coronary thrombosis Blood clot in a coronary artery usually leading to coronary artery narrowing.

Deep-vein thrombosis (DVT) Clots in the veins of the leg.

Defibrillator Equipment that delivers electric shocks to correct abnormal heart beats.

Diabetes Disease caused by lack of insulin, in which the body is unable to store sugar. May be treated with insulin, or diet and drugs.

Diastole Relaxation of the heart between beats when it is filling with blood.

Diastolic blood pressure (DBP) Lower of the two blood pressure readings taken when the heart is relaxing.

Digoxin Drug used to strengthen the heart and control atrial fibrillation.

Diuretic Water tablet that increases passage of fluid through the kidneys.

Doppler ultrasound Ultrasound technique used to study the speed and direction of blood flow. Sounds like a washing machine.

Dyspnoea Shortness of breath.

Echocardiography (Echo) Painless means of studying the heart's structure by bouncing ultrasound waves off the heart.

Ejection fraction (EF) Medical measure of the amount of blood pumped out of the left ventricle (pumping chamber) with each heart beat, usually over 50%.

Electrocardiogram (ECG or EKG) Recording of the electrical activity of the heart.

Electrophysiological study (EPS) Catheter test to evaluate the source of irregular heart beats and to judge the effect of treatments.

Embolus Blood clot which travels in the circulation. Can be in the vein or artery.

Endocarditis Infection inside the heart on a valve or the lining of the heart.

Endothelium Smooth inner lining of an artery.

Exercise test ('treadmill' test) ECG measures the heart's activity during exercise, usually on a treadmill. Used most often to diagnose coronary artery disease and assess its severity.

Fatty acids Chemical parts of triglycerides.

Fibrillation Erratic rapid contractions of the atria (atrial fibrillation) or ventricle (ventricular fibrillation). In ventricular fibrillation the heart stops.

Fibrinogen Blood thickening agent which occurs naturally in the body.

Flutter (atrial) A less erratic palpitation than atrial fibrillation.

Free radicals Damaging molecules produced by normal body processes such as breathing (oxygen) and digestion. Antioxidants reduce their effects.

Haemorrhage Bleeding.

Heart attack Death of heart muscle from lack of blood supply.

Heart block Slowing of the heart rate from an interrupted electrical circuit.

Heart failure Known medically as congestive heart failure(CHF) or congestive cardiac failure (CCF) When the heart cannot meet the body's demands usually because of heart muscle weakness. *See also* Congestive heart failure.

Heart–lung machine Machine that pumps blood to and from the body during heart surgery and keeps it full of oxygen.

Heredity Inherited by genetic means.

Hibernating myocardium Muscle which works but looks to be dead.

High blood pressure Serious increase in blood pressure.

High density lipoprotein (HDL) 'Good cholesterol' involved in removing cholesterol from the blood and blood vessels.

Holter monitor 24-hour ECG machine worn like a 'Walkman'.

Hypercholesterolaemia High cholesterol in the blood.

Hyperlipidaemia High fats in the blood.

Hypertension High blood pressure.

Hypotension Low blood pressure.

Hypoxia Lack of oxygen.

Immunosuppressive drugs Medication used to stop the body rejecting a transplant.

Incompetence Valve that is leaking.

Infarct Scar tissue with permanent damage to the heart muscle.

Ischaemia Inadequate blood supply usually caused by narrowed arteries. Ischaemic heart disease (IHD) is the consequence of ischaemia from narrowed coronary arteries.

Keloid Overgrowth of an operation scar.

Lipids Fats.

Lipoproteins Proteins, acting like taxis, carrying fats.

Low density lipoprotein (LDL) 'Bad cholesterol' which sticks to the artery walls.

Lumen Inside of a tube.

Mitral valve Valve between the left atrium and left ventricle.

Mitral valve prolapse (MVP) Floppy mitral valve causing one of the two leaflets to bulge backwards. This may cause a leak to occur but is often harmless.

Monounsaturated fat Healthy sort of fat found in olive oil and peanut oil. Can lower LDL cholesterol.

Mortality rate Number of deaths usually per year.

MRI *see* Nuclear magnetic resonance

Murmur Sound of blood flowing round, heard by a stethoscope. May be normal or point to disease. An echocardiogram will help diagnosis.

Myocardial biopsy Taking a sample of heart muscle.

Myocardial infarction (MI) Heart attack.

Myocardial ischaemia Reduced (poor) blood supply to the heart muscle.

Myocardium Heart muscle.

Necrosis Death of body tissue.

Nitroglycerin Drug used to relieve angina (e. g. glyceryl trinitrate – GTN).

Non-invasive Means of diagnosis or treatment without the need for an incision.

Nuclear magnetic resonance (NMR) Use of a magnetic field to take images of the heart and body. Also known as magnetic resonance imaging (MRI). NMR should not be undertaken if a pacemaker has been inserted but it can be used if a coronary stent is in place.

Obesity Being overweight. Medical definition is 20% above the average for your height and weight.

Occluded artery Totally blocked, may be acute or chronic.

Oedema Fluid usually in the lungs or round the ankles.

Open heart surgery Operation on the heart with the chest opened and a bypass machine used to pump the blood.

Pacemaker Small electrical device implanted surgically that regulates the heart beat usually preventing it going too slowly.

Palpitations Out of the ordinary heart beats. Can be rapid or missed or both.

Passive smoking Breathing in (and being poisoned by) someone else's cigarette smoke.

Percutaneous transluminal coronary angioplasty (PTCA) Long-winded term for angioplasty.

Pericarditis Inflammation of the pericardium.

Pericardium Smooth sac that surrounds the heart. When inflamed, it loses smoothness and becomes painful, leading to pericarditis.

Plaque Fatty deposits on the inner lining of an artery.

Platelets Small blood particles which stick together to form clots. Aspirin reduces their stickiness.

Polyunsaturated fat Fat in most vegetable oils which is liquid at room temperature. Tends to lower LDL cholesterol.

Positron emission tomography (PET) Imaging technique that tells us whether the heart muscle is alive and how it is functioning. A very expensive technique, so used sparingly.

Prophylaxis Anticipation and prevention, usually with drugs.

Pulmonary Relating to the lungs and breathing system.

Pulmonary valve Valve between the right ventricle and the pulmonary artery.

Regurgitation Leaking, e. g. mitral regurgitation – a leaking mitral valve.

Renal Relating to the kidneys.

Resuscitation Reviving someone who seems to be dead by heart massage and mouth-to-mouth breathing.

Risk factor Feature related to an increased chance of developing a disease (e. g. smoking and high cholesterol levels are risk factors for heart disease).

Saturated fat Animal fat, solid at room temperature. Increases total and LDL cholesterol.

Septum Muscle dividing the right from left side of the heart. A defect or hole in the heart is a 'septal defect'.

Sinus node (sinoatrial [SA] node) The heart's natural pacemaker or master switch.

Sodium Sodium chloride is the chemical name for salt.

Sphygmomanometer Machine to measure blood pressure.

Stenosis Narrowing.

Stent Metal cage inserted by a balloon into an artery, which, when expanded, holds an artery open. It is left in place. The balloon is removed.

Sternum Breastbone.

Stethoscope Instrument for listening to sounds in the body.

Streptokinase Clot-dissolving drug.

Stroke Damage to the brain as a result of interruption in the blood supply.

Syncope Sudden loss of consciousness.

Systole Heart contracting – pumping out blood.

Systolic blood pressure Highest pressure measured when the heart contracts and pumps out blood.

Tachycardia Rapid heart beat, typically over 100 beats per minute.

Thallium test Radioactive test to look at the extent of heart muscle damage (whether permanent or reversible).

Thrombolysis Breaking down blood clots – 'clot busting'.

Thrombosis Blood clot.

Tissue plasminogen activator (TPA) Clot-dissolving treatment.

Transoesophageal echocardiography (TOE) Specialized echo machine looking at the heart from inside the food pipe (oesophagus).

Transplant Heart replaced with one from someone else.

Triglycerides Fats used as energy source. High levels increase the risk for coronary disease.

Unsaturated fats Fats that are liquid or a soft solid at room temperature.

Vasodilator Drug that opens up (widens) arteries.

Vein Low pressure blood vessels carrying blood back to the heart to pick up oxygen.

Ventricle Heart muscle pump.

Ventricular septal defect Hole between the right and left ventricle.

Vitamin E Antioxidant vitamin found in vegetable oils, green leafy vegetables, wholegrain cereals, and almonds and hazelnuts.

Appendix 1

Practising what I preach!

What do you do, as a doctor, to prevent heart disease?

With this question, people are really asking whether we, as doctors, follow our own advice. Not often, is the honest answer, but here is what I do. First I have a family history, so I'm more concerned with prevention as a result. This is very important.

- I don't smoke.
- I avoid salt and salty foods.
- I take regular exercise, walking briskly 2 miles a day, four times a week. I avoid lifts and take the stairs.
- I watch my weight. I eat sensibly but not obsessionally (see Chapter 9). I try to keep my cholesterol at 5.0 mmol/litre with a good HDL (see the section on *Coronary artery disease and cholesterol* in Chapter 2).
- I enjoy wine.
- I have my blood pressure checked once a year.
- I try to stay calm!

What would you do if you had angina or a heart attack?

First I would be disappointed that I had not been able to prevent it.

- I'd have my cholesterol checked again.
- I would take aspirin and medications prescribed.
- I would want to know how I did on an exercise test and how my pump performed on an echocardiogram.

What drugs would you take?

Aspirin, statin, ACE inhibitor or AII antagonists. I have mild asthma so I probably could not tolerate a beta-blocker.

Would you have an angiogram done?

I would not hesitate to have an angiogram if this was recommended to determine the extent of the problem. I would want to look at it myself!

Would you have an angioplasty or surgery if recommended?

Again, I would have no hesitation to agree to whatever is appropriate. I would select my surgeon, cardiologist or anaesthetist carefully. I realize that I would have better information about this than a layman.

Would you return to your normal workload afterwards?

I would look carefully at my workload and almost certainly cut back on my commitments. I would try and reduce my hours, avoid committees and cut down lectures and on unnecessary travel. I would spend more time with my family, recognizing that I should have done this much sooner.

Do you think heart disease would affect you psychologically?

Yes. Like most doctors I have an unhealthy feeling of invincibility regarding my own health and it would shatter the myth! Being positive by nature would help me pick up the pieces, although I would have to recognize that those who 'told me so' were right.

Appendix 2

Useful addresses

If you write for information from any of these organizations, it is helpful to enclose a large self-addressed envelope. We have not included email numbers as these change frequently.

American Heart Association
7272 Greenville Avenue
Dallas
Texas TX 75321
Tel: 00 1 800 242 8721
Fax: 00 1 214-706-2139
Website: www.americanheart.org
Promotes healthier life styles by training volunteers throughout the USA.

ASH (Action on Smoking and Health)
102 Clifton Street
London EC2A 4HW
Helpline: 0800 169 0169
Tel: 020 7739 5902
Fax: 020 7613 0531
Website: www.ash.org.uk
National organization with local branches. Campaigns on antismoking policies. Offers free information on website or for sale from H.Q. Catalogue on request.

Association of Qualified Curative Hypnotherapists
PO Box 9989
Birmingham B14 4WA
Tel: 0121 6931223
Website: www.aqch.org
Professional membership body, offers information about hypnotherapy and list of registered practitioners.

Blood Pressure Association
60 Cranmer Terrace
London SW17 0QS
Tel: 020 8772 4994
Fax: 020 8772 4999
Website: www.bpassoc.org.uk
Offers information and fact sheets about high blood pressure and the various ways it can be treated. An SAE A4 size envelope requested with two first class stamps.

British Acupuncture Council
63 Jeddo Road
London W12 9HQ
Tel: 020 8735 0400
Fax: 020 8735 0404
Website: www.acupuncture.org.uk
Professional body offering lists of qualified acupuncture therapists.

British Dietetic Association
5th Floor
Charles House
148–149 Great Charles Street
Birmingham B3 3HT
Tel: 0121 200 8080
Fax: 0121 200 8081
Website: www.bda.uk.com
Professional association supporting dietitians.

British Heart Foundation
14 Fitzhardinge Street
London W1H 4DH
Helpline: 08450 708070
Tel: 020 7935 0185
Fax: 020 7486 5820
Website: www.bhf.org.uk
Funds research, promotes education and raises money to buy equipment to treat heart disease. HeartstartUK arranges training in emergency life-saving techniques. To contact local support groups tel. 020 7487 7110. Publications orderline 01604 640016.

**British Herbal Medicine
Association**
1 Wickham Road
Boscombe
Bournemouth BH7 6JX
Tel: 01202 433 691
Fax: 01202 417 079
Website: www.bhma.info
*Offers information, encourages
research and promotes high
quality standards. Advises
members on legalities for
importers, vets advertisements
and defends the right of the
public to choose herbal
medicines and be able to obtain
them freely.*

**British Holistic Medical
Association**
59 Lansdowne Place
Hove BN3 1FL
Tel: 01273 725 951
Fax: 01273 725 951
Website: www.bhma.org
*Promotes awareness of the
holistic approach to health
among practitioners and the
public through publications,
self-help tapes, conferences and
a network of local groups.*

**British Homeopathic
Association**
Hahnemann House
29 Park Street West
Luton LU1 3BE
Tel: 0870 444 3950
Fax: 0870 444 3960
Website: www.trusthomeopathy.org
*Professional body offering lists
of qualified homeopathic
practitioners.*

British Hypertension Society
BP Unit
St George's Hospital
Cranmer Terrace
London SW17 0RE
Tel: 020 8725 3412
Fax: 020 8725 2959
Website: www.bhsoc.org
*Professional body disseminating
guidelines to health care
professionals.*

**British Medical Acupuncture
Society**
12 Marbury House
Higher Whitley
Warrington WA4 4QW
Tel: 01925 730 727
Fax: 01925 730 492
Website:
www.medical-acupuncture.co.uk
*Professional body offering
training to doctors and list of
accredited acupuncture
practitioners.*

Cardiomyopathy Association
40 The Metro Centre
Tolpits Lane
Watford WD1 8SB
Helpline: 0800 0181 024
Tel: 01923 249977
Fax: 01923 249987
Website: www.cardiomyopathy.org
*Offers information for health
professionals; also support and
information for people with
cardiomyopathy and their
families.*

**Chest, Heart and Stroke
Association (N. Ireland)**
21 Dublin Road
Belfast BT2 7HB
Helpline: 08457 697 299
Tel: 02890 320 184
Fax: 02890 333 487
Website: www.nichsa.com
*Funds research and provides
information on chest, heart and
stroke-related illnesses.*

**Chest, Heart and Stroke
(Scotland)**
65 North Castle Street
Edinburgh EH2 3LT
Helpline: 0845 077 6000
Tel: 0131 225 6963
Fax: 0131 220 6313
Website: www.chss.org.uk
*Funds research and provides
information on chest, heart and
stroke-related illnesses.*

**Complementary Medical
Association**
67 Eagle Heights
The Falcons
Bramlands Close
London SW11 2LJ
Helpline: 0845 129 8434
Tel: 01424 438 801
Fax: 0845 129 8435
Website: www.the-cma.org.uk
*A not-for-profit medical body
offering membership to highly
qualified practitioners of
complementary medicine.
Has a database of accredited
practitioners around the UK.*

Consumers' Association
2 Marylebone Road
London NW1 4DF
Helpline: 0845 307 4000
Tel: 020 7770 7000
Fax: 020 7770 7600
Website: www.which.net
*Campaigns on behalf of
consumers and produces reports
on products including foods.
Publications order line:
0800 252100.*

Coronary Prevention Group (CPG)
London School of Hygiene &
Tropical Medicine
2 Taviton Street
London WC1H 0BT
Tel: 020 7927 2125
Fax: 020 7927 2127
Website: www.healthnet.org.uk
*First British charity devoted to
prevention of coronary heart
disease. Produces booklets and
fact sheets available on the
website or by post. Please send
SAE.*

Countryside Agency
John Dower House
Crescent Place
Cheltenham G50 3RA
Tel: 01242 521381
Fax: 01242 584270
Website: www.countryside.gov.uk
*Working with other agencies,
identifies problems and develops
solutions to economic,
environmental and community
issues for the enjoyment of the
countryside.*

Department of Health (DoH)
PO Box 777
London SE1 6XH
Helpline: 0800 555 777
Tel: 020 7210 4850
Fax: 01623 724 524
Textphone: 020 7210 5025
Website: www.doh.gov.uk
*Produces literature about health
issues, available via helpline.
A more technical site with
National Service Frameworks
available from internet e.g.*
www.doh.gov.uk/nsf/bloodpressure

Diabetes UK
10 Parkway
London NW1 7AA
Helpline: 020 7424 1030
Tel: 020 7424 1000
Textline 020 7424 1031
Fax: 020 7424 1001
Website: www.diabetes.org.uk
*Provides advice and
information on diabetes;
has local support groups.*

**Drinkline (National Alcohol
Helpline)**
Helpline: 0800 917 8282
*Funded by Dept. of Health,
provides educational material
for schools, health professionals
and general information on
drink, sex and drugs issues.
Refers to local agencies for
support.*

Health Development Agency
Holborn Gate
330 High Holborn
London WC1V 7BA
Helpline: 0870 121 4194
Tel: 020 7430 0850
Fax: 020 7061 3390
Website: www.hda-online.org.uk
*Formerly Health Education
Authority; now only deals with
research. Publications on health
matters can be ordered on
0800 555 777.*

Health Which?
PO Box 44
Hertford X SG14 1LH
Tel: 0800 252100
Fax: 0845 3074001
Website: www.which.net
*Requests for any Consumer
Association (Which?)
publications, can be ordered
here.*

Heart UK
7 North Road
Maidenhead SL6 1PE
Tel: 01628 628 638
Fax: 01628 628 698
Website: www.heartuk.org.uk
*Offers information, advice and
support to people with coronary
heart disease and especially to
those at high risk of familial
hyper- cholesterolaemia.
Members receive bimonthly
magazine.*

**Institute for Complementary
Medicine**
PO Box 194
London SE16 7QZ
Tel: 020 7237 5165
Fax: 020 7237 5175
Website: www.icmedicine.co.uk
*Umbrella group for
complementary medicine
organizations. Offers informed,
safe choice to public, British
register of practitioners and
refers to accredited training
courses. S.a.e. requested for
information.*

Irish Heart Foundation
4 Clyde Road
Ballsbridge
Dublin 4
Tel: 00 353 1 668 5001
Fax: 00 353 1 668 5896
Website: www.irishheart.ie
*Offers information,
publications, training and
support in prevention of heart
disease. Collaborates with other
heart-related organizations and
has some local support groups.*

**National Institute
of Medical Herbalists**
56 Longbrook Street
Exeter EX4 6AH
Tel: 01392 426 022
Fax: 01392 498 963
Website: www.nimh.org.uk
*Professional body representing
qualified, practising medical
herbalists. Offer lists of
accredited medical herbalists.
S.A.E. requested.*

**NHS Direct (England,
Northern Ireland & Wales)**
Helpline: 0845 4647
Tel: 020 8867 1367
Textphone 0845 606 4647
Website: www.nhsdirect.nhs.uk
*NHS Direct is a 24 hour helpline
offering confidential healthcare
advice, information and referral
service 365 days of the year. A
good first port of call for any
health advice.*

NHS Health Scotland
Woodburn House
Canaan Lane
Edinburgh EH10 4SG
Tel: 0131 536 5500
Fax: 0131 536 5501
Textphone 0131 536 5503
Website: www.healthscotland.com
*NHS health education board for
Scotland publishing leaflets on a
variety of health issues.*

NHS Scotland 0800 224 488

**Quit (National Society
for Non-Smokers)**
211 Old Street
London EC1V 9NR
Helpline: 0800 002200
Tel: 020 7251 1551
Fax: 020 7251 1661
Website: www.quit.org.uk
*Offers advice to stop smoking
in English & Asian languages;
also to schools, and on
pregnancy. Runs training
courses for health professionals.
Can put people in touch with
local support groups.*

Resuscitation Council
5th Floor,
Tavistock House North
Tavistock Square
London WC1H 9HR
Tel: 020 7388 4678
Fax: 020 7383 0773
Website: www.resus.org.uk
*Sets standards and runs courses
on resuscitation for health care
professionals. Funds research.*

Royal Life Saving Society UK
River House, High Street
Broom B50 4HN
Tel: 01789 773994
Fax: 01789 773995
Website: www.lifesavers.org.uk
*Leading organization promoting
prevention of drowning through
training and activities in
life-saving techniques.*

**Scottish Heart and Arterial
Disease Risk Prevention
(SHARP)**
Department of Medicine and
Therapeutics
Ninewells Hospital and Medical
School
Dundee DD1 9SY
Tel: 01382 660111
Fax: 01382 660675
Website: www.heartscotland.org
*Charity run by health
professionals aiming, through
scientific meetings and research,
to reduce incidence of
cardiovascular disease in
Scotland. Produces guidelines
for health professionals, leaflets
and videos for their patients.*

Sexual Dysfunction Association
PO Box 10296
London SW17 9WH
Helpline: 020 8767 7791
Website: www.impotence.org.uk
*Gives advice on sexual problems,
such as erectile dysfunction.*

Society of Homeopaths
4a Artizan Road
Northampton NN1 4HU
Tel: 01604 621 400
Fax: 01604 622 622
Website: www.homeopathy-soh.org
*Professional body, offers lists
of accredited homeopathic
therapists and free general
information.*

Sport England
3rd Floor
Victoria House
Bloomsbury Square
London WC1B 4SE
Tel: 020 7273 1500
Fax: 020 7273 1868
Website: www.sportengland.org
*Government agency promoting
sport in England with a wide
variety of activity programmes
in order to foster a healthier
lifestyle.*

St John Ambulance
27 St John's Lane
London EC1M 4BU
Helpline: 08700 104 950
Tel: 08702 355 231
Fax: 08700 104 065
Website: www.sja.org.uk
*Provides first aid training for
adults and young people and
cover for events. Has a fleet of
ambulances and provides
services to homeless people and
library services to hospitals.*

Stroke Association
Stroke House
240 City Road
London EC1V 2PR
Helpline: 0845 303 3100
Tel: 020 7566 0300
Fax: 020 7490 2686
Website: www.stroke.org.uk
*Funds research and provides
information now specializing
in stroke only. Publications can
be ordered from 01604 623 933.*

**Vegetarian Society of the
United Kingdom**
Parkdale
Dunham Road
Altrincham WA14 4QG
Tel: 0161 925 2000
Fax: 0161 926 9182
Website: www.vegsoc.org
*Offers information on the
vegetarian way of life, day and
residential training courses at
own Centre. Provides literature
for GCSE projects, advice to
school caterers. Food
manufacturers and restaurants
can apply for vegetarian
accreditation.*

Women's Health
52 Featherstone Street
London EC1Y 8RT
Helpline: 0845 125 5254
Tel: 020 7251 6333
Fax: 020 7250 4152
Minicom: 020 7490 5489
Website:
www.womenshealthlondon.org.uk
*Provides information on
gynaecological and sexual issues
to help women make informed
decisions about their health.
Range of publications and
quarterly newsletter. To use
reference library, please
telephone first.*

**Women's Health Concern
(WHC)**
PO Box 2126
Marlow SL7 2RY
Helpline: 01628 483 612
Tel: 01628 488 065
Fax: 01628 474 042
Website:
www.womens-health-concern.org
*National charity that offers help
to women, particularly on
questions of hormone health,
HRT and gynaecology. Request
S.A.E. for information.
Website for menopause queries:*
www.menopausematters.co.uk

Appendix 3

Useful publications and alert systems

Books

High Blood Pressure – the 'at your fingertips' guide (3rd edition), by
Dr Tom Fahey, Professor Deirdre Murphy with Dr Julian Tudor Hart,
published by Class Publishing (2004). ISBN 1 85959 090 X.

Diabetes – the 'at your fingertips' guide (5th edition) by Professor
Peter Sönksen, Dr Charles Fox and Sue Judd, published by Class
Publishing (2003). ISBN 1 85959 087 X.

Stop that heart attack! (3rd edition), by Dr Derrick Cutting, published
by Class Publishing (2004). ISBN 1 85959 096 9.

General booklets

The **British Heart Foundation** publishes many excellent and recently
revised booklets on all aspects of heart disease, including *Women
and heart disease; Smoking and your heart; Implantable
cardioverter defibrillators; Trim the fat from your diet; Put your
heart into walking*. Head office and regional addresses can be found
in Appendix 2.

In Scotland, the **SHARP programme** is an excellent source of
information – information is available online at
http://www.dundee.ac.uk/sharp/

The **Family Doctor Series** covers around 27 titles including
cholesterol, stress and high blood pressure; individual booklets are
priced very cheaply. Published by FDP, 10 Butchers Row, Banbury,
Oxon OX16 8JH, Tel: 01295 276627.

Ask your doctor for free leaflets that may have been provided by drug
companies, and also from local NHS Trusts etc.

The **Coronary Prevention Group** (address in Appendix 2) provides good advice. Look on their website for further information.
Diabetes UK publishes a leaflet on *Eating well with diabetes*, which should be useful for people with diabetes and heart problems.
In America, it is difficult to beat the booklets from the **American Heart Association** (address in Appendix 2). Website address: http://www.americanheart.org/ – many publications listed are listed on their website, including *To Your Health! A Guide to Heart-Smart Living; Fitting in Fitness; 365 Ways to Get Out the Fat: A Tip a Day to Trim the Fat Away* and *6 Weeks to Get Out the FAT.*

Food and cooking

There are many books on healthy foods with sample menus:
The Light-Hearted Cookbook: Recipes for a Healthy Heart, by Anne Lindsay, published by Grub Street/British Heart Foundation (1999), ISBN 1 902304 15 2.
The Everyday Light-Hearted Cookbook, by Anne Lindsay, published by Grub Street/British Heart Foundation (1994), ISBN 0 948817 78 X.
Help your heart: a practical guide with recipes by Jill Davies and Claire Dickerson, published by Smith Gordon & Co. (1992). ISBN 1 854630 44 X.
Which? way to a healthier diet by Judy Byrne, published by the Consumers' Association/Hodder Headline (1993). ISBN 0 340591 0 13.
Healthy eating on a plate by Janette Marshall, published by Vermilion (1995). ISBN 0 091808 57 X.
Cooking for a healthy heart by Jacqui Lynas, published by Hamlyn/Heart UK (2004). ISBN 0 600610 51 9.

Stopping smoking

How to Stop Smoking and Stay Stopped for Good, by Gillian Riley, published by Vermilion (2003). ISBN 0 09 188776 3.
Stop Smoking in Five Days by Judy Perlmutter, published by HarperCollins (1997). ISBN 0 722535 83 X.
Allen Carr's Easy Way to Stop Smoking, by Allen Carr, published by Penguin (1999). ISBN 0 14 027763 3.
Stop Smoking for Good, by Robert Brynin, published by Hodder & Stoughton (1995). ISBN 0 340 63240 2.

Appendix 4

This is just a guide. A more accurate assessment is provided in Figure 9.1

Height to weight – adults (desirable)

Height in flat shoes		Average weight in pounds and kilograms (in indoor clothing)					
		17–19 yr		20–24 yr		25–29 yr	
cm	ft in	kg	st lb	kg	st lb	kg	st lb
MEN							
157.5	5 2	54.0	8 7	58.1	9 0	60.8	9 7
160.0	5 3	55.8	8 11	59.9	9 6	62.6	9 11
162.6	5 4	57.6	9 1	61.7	9 10	64.0	10 1
165.1	5 5	59.4	9 4	63.0	9 13	65.3	10 4
167.6	5 6	61.2	9 8	64.4	10 1	67.1	10 7
170.2	5 7	63.0	9 13	65.8	10 4	68.5	10 11
172.7	5 8	64.9	10 3	67.6	10 8	70.3	11 1
175.3	5 9	66.7	10 7	69.4	10 13	72.1	11 4
177.8	5 10	68.5	10 11	71.2	11 3	73.9	11 8
180.3	5 11	70.3	11 1	73.0	11 7	75.8	11 13
182.9	6 0	72.6	11 6	75.3	11 11	78.0	12 4
185.4	6 1	74.4	11 10	77.1	12 1	80.3	12 8
188.0	6 2	76.2	12 0	78.9	12 6	82.6	13 0
190.5	6 3	78.0	12 4	80.8	12 10	84.4	13 4
193.0	6 4	79.8	12 8	82.1	12 13	86.2	13 8
WOMEN							
147.3	4 10	44.9	7 1	46.3	7 4	48.5	7 8
149.9	4 11	46.3	7 4	47.6	7 7	49.9	7 11
152.4	5 0	47.6	7 7	49.0	7 10	51.3	8 1
154.9	5 1	49.4	7 11	50.8	8 0	52.6	8 4
157.5	5 2	51.3	8 1	52.2	8 3	54.0	8 7
160.0	5 3	52.6	8 4	53.5	8 6	55.3	8 10
162.6	5 4	54.4	8 8	54.9	8 8	56.7	8 13
165.1	5 5	56.2	8 11	56.7	8 13	58.5	9 3
167.6	5 6	57.6	9 1	58.5	9 3	60.3	9 7
170.2	5 7	59.0	9 4	59.9	9 6	61.7	9 10
172.7	5 8	60.8	9 7	61.7	9 10	63.5	10 0
175.3	5 9	62.6	9 11	63.5	10 0	65.3	10 4
177.8	5 10	64.4	10 1	65.3	10 4	67.1	10 7
180.3	5 11	66.7	10 7	67.6	10 8	69.4	10 13
182.9	6 0	68.9	10 11	69.9	11 0	71.7	11 4

30–39 yr			40–49 yr			50–59 yr			60–69yr		
kg	st	lb	kg	st	lb	kg	st	lb	kg	st	lb
62.1	9	11	63.5	10	0	64.4	10	1	63.0	9	13
64.0	10	1	65.3	10	4	65.8	10	4	64.4	10	1
65.8	10	4	67.1	10	8	67.6	10	8	66.2	10	6
67.6	10	8	68.9	10	11	69.4	10	13	68.0	10	10
69.4	10	13	70.8	11	1	71.2	11	3	69.9	11	0
71.2	11	3	73.0	11	7	73.5	11	8	72.1	11	4
73.0	11	7	74.8	11	11	75.3	11	11	73.9	11	8
74.8	11	11	76.7	12	1	77.1	12	1	76.2	12	0
77.1	12	1	78.9	12	6	79.4	12	7	78.5	12	4
78.9	12	6	80.8	12	10	81.6	12	11	80.8	12	7
81.2	12	11	83.0	13	1	83.9	13	3	83.0	13	1
83.0	13	1	84.8	13	4	85.7	13	7	85.3	13	6
85.3	13	6	87.1	13	10	88.0	13	11	87.5	13	11
87.5	13	11	89.4	14	1	90.3	14	3	89.8	14	1
90.3	14	3	92.1	14	7	93.0	14	8	92.5	14	7
52.2	8	3	55.3	8	10	56.7	8	13	57.6	9	1
53.1	8	4	56.2	8	11	57.6	9	1	58.5	9	3
54.4	8	7	57.6	9	1	59.0	9	4	59.4	9	4
55.8	8	11	59.0	9	4	60.3	9	7	60.8	9	7
57.2	9	0	60.3	9	7	61.7	9	10	62.1	9	11
58.5	9	3	61.7	9	10	63.5	10	0	64.0	10	1
59.9	9	6	63.5	10	0	65.3	10	4	65.8	10	4
61.2	9	8	64.9	10	3	67.1	10	8	67.6	10	8
63.0	9	13	66.7	10	7	68.9	10	11	69.4	10	13
64.4	10	1	68.5	10	11	70.8	11	4	71.2	11	3
66.2	10	6	70.3	11	1	72.6	11	6	73.0	11	7
68.0	10	10	72.1	11	4	74.4	11	10	74.8	11	11
69.9	11	0	74.4	11	10	76.7	12	1	–		–
72.1	11	4	76.7	12	1	78.9	12	6	–		–
74.4	11	10	78.9	12	6	81.6	12	11	–		–

Index

NOTE: the index covers pages
1–287. Page numbers in italics
refer to diagrams and tables;
g refers to glossary. **Bold** is used
to highlight emergency situations.

Accupro (quinapril) *39*
ACE (angiotensin-converting
    enzyme) inhibitors *38–9, 41,*
    42–3, 131, 280*g*
  and diuretics *168,* 171
  in heart attack 140, 141
  in heart failure 160, 173–4
acebutolol (Sectral) *38, 92*
Acepril (captopril) *38,* 42
acupuncture 20–1, 126
Adalat LA (nifedipine) *38, 92*
Adalat (nifedipine) *38,* 42, *92,* 99
Adizem (diltiazem) *38,* 42, *92,* 99
adrenal glands 29
adrenaline 29–30, 41, 181, 188
age
  blood pressure 27–8, 31
  digoxin medication 188
  exercise 269
  and gender in coronary heart
    disease 67–8
  heart failure incidence 157
  heart transplantation 174
  palpitations 182, 184

  risk in older people *12,* 31–2,
    33, 36–7
  sexual activity 214
  and smoking 17
  thrombolysis (clot buster
    medication) 139
  work after bypass surgery 124
AICD (automatic implantable
    cardioverter defibrillator)
    200, 280*g*
alcohol 246–8
  atrial fibrillation 191
  calorie content 262
  and depression 147
  heart failure 158
  with medication 103, 172
  palpitations 179, 184
  and smoking 19
  with warfarin 172
Aldactide 41
Aldactone (spironolactone) *38,*
    41
Aldomet 44 (methyldopa) 44
Alkaseltzer 92
alpha-blockers *39, 41,* 43
alternative therapies *see*
    complementary therapies
ambulance (999) 137–8
Amias (candesartan) *39*
amiloride *38,* 41, *168*

amiodarone 188, 189, 193
amlodipine (Istin) *38*, 42, *92*, 99,
220
anaemia 29, 75, 159–60, 163, 181
causing blackout 201
anaesthetic
general 117, 194, 195
local 86, 88, 104, 105, 166, 175
EPS test 187
insertion of pacemakers 197
mitral valvuloplasty 208
aneurysm 169, 280*g*
anger 64, 76, 136, 145–6
angina 4, 12, 42, 43, 47, 280*g*
after meals 81
cause 75–6, 136
different from heart attack
78–9, *79*, 136
driving 81, 1112
emergency action 80, 148
felt as indigestion 135
medication 93, 101–3
pain despite medication 79–80
preventing return after surgery
124–5, 131
self-help 91
sexual activity 214, 216, 219
symptoms 76–81, *77*
Syndrome X 90–1
treatment
alternative therapies 125–30
medical 91–103
surgical 104–25
unstable 79, 111
in valvular disease 205
angiogram 81, 280*g*
after heart attack 145
hospital procedure 85–7, 88–90
results 89

Syndrome X 90–1
angioplasty 85, 91, 280*g*, 285*g*
after heart attack 145
alternative to clot buster drugs
149
choice of procedure 110–11
complications 107, 111
continuation of medication
111–12
duration of effects 106–7,
111–12
in older people 139
procedure 104–5, *106*, 107
when not recommended 107–8
see also mitral valvuloplasty
angiotensin II antagonists *39*, *41*,
42–3, 46, 131, 141
heart failure *168*, 171, 173
angiotensin converting enzyme
inhibitors *see* ACE
ankle swelling *41*, 42, 99–100, 160,
162, 169
antacids *79*
antibiotics 209
anticoagulant 280*g*
see alslo heparin; warfarin
antioxidants 51, 53, 127, 280*g*
anxiety 178–9, 215–16
aorta 3, *3*, 5, *6*, *176*, 280*g*
in bypass surgery 113, *114*
cardiac catheterization 104
see also palpitations
aortic valve 5, *6*, 7, 75, 280*g*
incompetence/stenosis 204
aporphine (Uprima) 221
appetite loss 147, 170, 188
Aprinox (bendrofluazide) *38*, 40
Aprovel (irbestartan) *39*
arm pain 76, 134–5, *134*

arrhythmia 280*g*
  see also palpitations
arteries 280*g*
  muscles 27, *28*
  narrowing/blocking 4, *28*, 48, 56
  spasm through illegal drugs *66*,
    67
  see also coronary artery bypass
    graft; coronary heart
    disease; *individual arteries*
arthritis pills 173
ASD *see* atrial septal defect
aspirin 80, 88, 91–2, 101, 111
  in heart attack emergency
    137, 149
  instead of warfarin 172
  to prevent pain recurrence 131,
    140, 141
asthma 42, 99
atenolol (Tenormin, Totamol) *38*,
  41, *92*, 96, 97, 140
atenolol + chlorthalidone
  (Tenoret 50, Tenoretic) *39*
atenolol + nifedipine (Tenif,
  Beta-Adalat) *39*
atheroma 11–12, 75, 280*g*
  see also coronary artery disease
atherosclerosis 11
  see also coronary heart disease
atorvastatin (Lipitor) *58*
atria, left/right 5–6, *6*, *176*, 190,
  199, 280*g*
atrial fibrillation 160, 170, 172,
  184, 280*g*, 283*g*
  causes 190–1
  defibrillators 200
  tests 192
  treatment 191–5, 192–5
  what it is 189–90, 191

  see also palpitations
atrial septal defect (ASD) 7, 281*g*,
  286*g*
atrioventricular (AV) node 8, *9*,
  190, 281*g*
automatic implantable
  cardioverter defibrillator
  (AICD) 200, 280*g*

bacterial endocarditis 209–10,
  283*g*
balloon treatment *see* angioplasty; mitral valvuloplasty;
  stent
bananas 243
Baratol (indoramin) *39*
batteries for pacemakers 198
beer *see* alcohol
bendrofluazide (Aprinox) *38*, 40,
  168
bendrofluazide + propranolol
  (Inderetic) *39*
Benecol 234
beta carotene 53, 125
Beta-Adalat (atenolol +
  nifedipine) *39*
beta-blockers *38*, 41–2, *41*, 48, *92*,
  281*g*
  with amlodipine/felodipine/
    nifedipine 99
  for angina 95–6, 131
  best time to take 98, 102
  danger of suddenly stopping
    treatment 97, 98, 100
  in heart attack 140, 141
  heart failure *168*, 173
  hydrophilic/lipophilic types 97
  instead of calcium antagonists
    100

with nitrates 98
for palpitations 187–8
running out of tablets 98, 102
side effects 96–7
Betaloc (metoprolol) *38*, 41, *92*
Beta-Prograne (propranolol) *38*,
    92,
Betim (timolol) *38*, *92*
bezafibrate (Bezalip) *58*
Biocadren (timolol) *38*
biopsy 175, 281*g*, 285*g*
birth *see* heredity
bisoprolol (Emcor, Monocor) *38*,
    41, *92*, 96, 140, *168*
blackouts 10, 201–2, 205
bloating sensation *41*, *58*
Blocadren (timolol) *92*
blood *see* blood circulation; blood
    clotting; blood group; blood
    pressure; blood vessels;
    cholesterol; oxygen; thinning
    of blood; valves of heart
blood circulation process 1–4, *6*
blood clotting 4, 15, 72, 281*g*
    in narrowed artery 78, 133
    platelets 285*g*
    thrombolysis 149
    warfarin medication 87–8, 172
    see also aspirin; clot buster
        drugs; gingko; plaque
blood group in transplantation
    175
blood pressure 281*g*
    diastolic/systolic 27, *28*, 35–6
    fluctuations 30
    high insulin levels 65–6
    home monitoring machines 34
    how it works 27–8
    lowering of 95, 127

measurement 8, 27, 30, 31, 34–6,
    35
nicotine replacement problem
    23
raised/high 4, 12, 27–8, *28*, 284*g*
    angina 75
    atrial fibrillation 190
    cause 29
    danger of not treating 47
    in heart failure 158
    'rebound effect' 45, 148
    risks 27–8
    'rule of halves' *32*, 33–4
    treatment 40–8
        see also side effects
    'white coat hypertension' 31
    salt 240, 242
    self-help 36–7
    specific risk factors 33
    tests 29
blood sugar levels 65–6
    see also diabetes
blood vessels 281*g*
    see also individual vessels,
        e.g. coronary arteries
Body Mass Index 252–4
brachial artery 36, 104, 281*g*
bradycardia 196, 281*g*
brain 5, *41*, 44
    see also cerebral
bread *232–3*, 234, 238, *241*
breast bone 76, 120, *134*
breast cancer 69–70, 71
breathing machine 118
breathlessness 10, 45, 96, 135,
    169, 283*g*
    in heart failure 161
bronchial tubes 118
bruising after angiogram 89–90

bumetanide *168*, 169
bundles, left/right 8, *9*, 281*g*
buproprion (Zyban) 26
bypass surgery 107
  blood vessels used 113, *114*, 115
  see mainly coronary artery
    bypass graft

CABG *see* coronary artery bypass
  graft
CAD *see* coronary artery disease
caffeine 179–80, 188, *243*, 246
calcium antagonists/blockers *38*,
  41, 42, 43, 90, *92*, 281*g*
  for atrial fibrillation 193
  with beta-blockers 99
  how they work 98–9
  with nitrates 99
  for palpitations 188
calories and joules 239, *244*,
  260–2, 269
candesartan (Amias) *39*, 131, *168*,
  171
cannabis 66–7
Capoten (captopril) *38*, 42
captopril (Capoten, Acepril) *38*,
  42, 140, *168*
captopril + hydrochlorothiazide
  (Capozide, Acezide) *39*
Carace (lisinopril) *38*, 42
carbon atoms 50–1
carbon dioxide 1
carbon monoxide 14–15, 66
Cardene SR (nicardipine) *38*, *92*
cardiac *see also* heart
cardiac ablation 192, 195, 281*g*
Cardilate MR (nifedipine) *38*, *92*
cardiologist 81, 104, 115, 195, 209,
  281*g*

cardiomemo machine 186–7
cardiomyopathy (hypertrophic/
  congestive) 158–9, 282*g*
cardiomyoplasty 177
cardiopulmonary bypass *see*
  heart-lung machine
cardioversion (electric shock
  treatment) 192–5, *194*, 196,
  282*g*
  versus pacemaker 196
Cardura (doxazosin) *39*, 43
carotid arteries 282*g*
carotid sinus massage (CSM) 183
carvedilol (Eucardic) *38*, *168*
catheterization, cardiac 81, 85, 86,
  104, 192
catheters 85
  cardiac catheter 81, 85, 86, 104,
    192, 281*g*
  guide catheter 104–5, *106*
  pacemaker 187, 195
  see also angiogram, coronary
CCU *see* coronary care unit
Celectol (celiprolol) *38*
celiprolol (Celectol) *38*
cephalic vein 197
cereals *236*, 240, *241*, *247*
cerebral embolism 282*g*
cerebral haemorrhage 282*g*
cerebral thrombosis 282*g*
chelation therapy warning 130
chemist *see* pharmacist advice
chest/heart pain 10, 45, 47, 76–8,
  77
  after bypass operation 119
  after recovery from heart attack
    145
  angina different from heart
    attack 136

in cardiac catheterization 104,
105
characteristics *79*
danger of rebound 97, 98
possible causes 78
site and radiation 134–5, *134*
see also angina; electrocardiogram; heart attack
chewing-gum 19
children
exposure to passive smoking 14
guilt feelings/self-blame 146
illegal drugs 67
visiting CCU 140
see also heredity
chlorthalidone (Hygroton) *38*, 40
chlorthalidone + atenolol
(Tenoret 50, Tenoretic) *39*
cholesterol 11, 49, 56–7, 225, 282*g*
after heart attack 155
facts and figures 48–9
ideal measurement 49–50, 60,
124, 155
lipid profile 48, 56–7, 73
lowering levels 59–60, 127
nicotinic acid 235
risks of high levels 4, 12, 49–54
self-help 55–7
self-testing kits 56
treatment 57–60, *58*
duration 59
side effects 57–8, *58*
when statins are indicated 173
see also fats; HDL; LDL
cholestyramine (Questran) *58*
Cialis (sildenafil) 220, 221
cigarettes *see* smoking
cigars *see* smoking, cigars
cilazapril (Vascace) *38, 168*

ciprofibrate (Modalim) *58*
circumflex artery *3, 114*
claudication 282*g*
see also leg pain
clopidogrel (Plavix) 88, 92, 111,
131, 141, 172
see also aspirin
clot buster drugs 139, 148–9
clotting of blood *see* blood
clotting
see also aspirin; clot buster
drugs; gingko; plaque
Co Aprovel (irbesartan + hydrochlorothiazide) *39*
co-proxamol 119
cocaine ('crack') 67
coffee *see* caffeine
cold remedies and angina tablets
102
coldness in hands and feet *41*, 96
collar bone 197
collaterals (enlarging arteries)
115, *116*, 282*g*
complementary therapies 125–30
cautionary advice 128–9
importance of labelling 128
medical scepticism 129
possibility of harm 130
training of practitioners 129
see also individual therapies,
e.g. acupuncture
concentration loss *41*, 45, 96,
118–19
after heart attack 147
conduction system 282*g*
see also heart, 'electrics'
congenital heart disease 9–10,
282*g*
congestive cardiomyopathy 158

constipation *41*, 42, *58*, 100, 119,
    237
contraceptive pill 16, 69
Coracten XL (nifedipine) *38*, *92*
Cordilox (verapamil) *38*, 42, *92*, 99
Corgard (nadolol) *92*
coronary angiogram
    see angiogram
coronary artery(ies) 1–4, *3*, *6*, 282*g*
    blocking/narrowing 9, 11–12,
        13, 15, *87*
    angina 136
    collaterals 115, *116*
    minor heart attack 136–7
    raised cholesterol 48–9
    relative risks *87*, 116–17
coronary artery bypass graft
    (CABG) 113–14, 282*g*
    'doing your own' (collaterals)
        115, *116*
    duration of success 117, 121
    intensive care 118
    possible post-operative
        problems 121
    post-operative posture 119
    preparation procedure 117
    procedure 113–14, *114*, 120
    reasons for choice 113, 116–17
    recovery period 119–22
    rehabilitation 122–3
        preventing return of angina
            124–5
    scarring 120–1
    transfer to normal ward 118–19
    wire stitches 120, 123
    see also heart transplant
coronary artery disease 11–13,
    282*g*
    cause of angina 75–6

illegal drugs 66–7
risk factors 12–13
and smoking 14
see also angina; angiogram;
    angioplasty; electrocardio-
    gram; heart attack; heart
    failure
coronary care unit (CCU) 138,
    140–1
coronary heart disease 32–3, *32*
    atrial fibrillation 191
    in women 67–74
    see also angina
coronary thrombosis 282*g*
cough, dry *41*, 42, 43, 171201
Coversyl (perindopril) *39*
Coversyl Plus (perindopril + inda-
    pamide) *39*
Cozaar (losartan) *39*, 42
Cozaar-Comp (losartan + hydro-
    chlorothiazide) *39*
'crack' *see* cocaine
cramps (muscular) *41*
Crestor (rosuvastatin) *58*
CSM *see* carotid sinus massage
cut-down technique (in angio-
    gram) 87, 90

dairy products 231, *232*
death 2, 4, 116–17
    of heart muscle 132
    and smoking 14
deep-vein thrombosis (DVT) 282*g*
    see also clotting of blood
defibrillator machine 194, 200,
    282*g*
dehydration 162
dental care 117
depression *41*, 96, 147, 215

diabetes *12*, 65–6, 282*g*
  nicotine replacements 23
  raised blood pressure 40, 41–2
diastole/diastolic pressure 7, 8,
    282*g*, 283*g*
diazepam (Diazemuls, Valium)
    105
diet 225–6
  after heart attack 140, 154–6
  Asian type 257, 259
  caffeine 179–80
  cooking methods 235–6, 238–9
  drinks 246–8
  eating out 258–9
  exercise after meals 152
  food labels 243–6, *247*
  food types 226–33, *232–3*
  guide to healthy eating *232–3*
  guidelines for daily intake
      244–5, 262–3
  health foods 52–4
  high blood pressure 37, 39, 155
  loss of appetite 147, 170
  lowering cholesterol 55
  meaning of 'portion' 261
  pain after eating 81
  snacks 243, 248–9, 263
  sodium levels *241–2*
  weight reduction 21, 249–63
  see also calories and joules;
      fats; fibre; fish; *individual
      foods*; oils; salt; sugar
dietitians 155
digoxin 40, 130, *168*, 283*g*
  atrial fibrillation 193, 206
  heart failure 170, 173, 193
  palpitations 188
diltiazem (Tildiem, Adizem,
    Dilzem) *38*, 42, *92*, 99, 102

Dilzem (diltiazem) *38*, 42, *92*, 99
Diovan (valsartan) *39*, 42
disopyramide 189, 193
diuretics *38*, 40–1, *41*, 100, 127,
    283*g*
  dehydration problem 162
  failure to work 170
  heart failure *168*, 173
  how they work 169–70
  low potassium level 183–4
  medication for heart attack 139,
      148
dizziness *41*, 95, 181
doctor *see* cardiologist; general
    practitioner
Doppler ultrasound 165, 283*g*
Dosette pill box 102
double bind trial 126
doxazosin (Cardura) *39*, 43
drinks, non-alcoholic 240, *242*,
    246
driving 81, 112, 123, 198
drowsiness *41*
drugs
  acting on brain *41*
  affecting blood pressure 29
  for angina *92*, 131
  causing sexual problems 217–18
  cholesterol-lowering 58–60, *58*
  clot buster 139, 148–9
  double blind trials 126
  heart attack 140–2
  heart failure *168*
  illegal 66–7
  metabolic agents 103
  names (generic and trade) 40
  nicotine addiction 14–15
  nicotine replacement side
      effects 23–4

palpitations 188–9
raised blood pressure *38–9*,
    40–4, *41*
reacting with Viagra 219
for smoking 26
suppressing new heart rejection
    175, 284*g*
vasodilator 287*g*
weight loss tablets 251
see also specific drugs
DVT *see* deep-vein thrombosis
Dyazide 41
dye injections in surgical
    procedures 85, 86, 88, 105
dyspnoea *see* breathlessness
Dytac 41

ECG *see* electrocardiogram
echocardiography 159, 163,
    164–6, *165*, 283*g*
in diagnosis of atrial fibrillation
    192
transoesophageal (TOE/TEE)
    287*g*
valvular heart disease 205–6
Ecstasy tablets 67
ED *see* erectile dysfunction
eggs 55, *232*, 234, *241*
ejection fraction (EF) 283*g*
EKG *see* electrocardiogram
Elantan (isosorbide mononitrate)
    92, 95
electrocardiogram (ECG) 81,
    82–4, *82–3*, 283*g*
diagnosis of atrial fibrillation
    192
diagnosis of heart attack 139
mobile recorder (Holter) 185–6,
    186, 284*g*

palpitations 181, 185–7
and sexual activity 213
'treadmill' test 83, 283*g*
electrolyte level in blood 170
electrophysiological tests (EPS)
    187, 192, 195, 283*g*
embolus 283*g*
see also clotting of blood
Emcor (bisoprolol) *38*, *92*
emergency situations
heart attack 135, 137–8, 148
prolonged angina pain 80, 148–9
emotions affecting heart 64, 65,
    76
after heart attack 145–7
employment *see* work
enalapril (Innovace) *39*, 42, 140,
    168
enalapril + hydrochlorothiazide
    (Innozide) *39*
endocarditis *see* bacterial endo-
    carditis
endothelium 4, 15, 283*g*
enzymes 139, 220, 281*g*
epilepsy 201
EPS *see* electrophysiological tests
erectile dysfunction (ED) *41*, 45,
    97–8, 216–21
warning of heart attack 135–6
Eucardic (glyceryl trinitrate) *38*
evidence-based medicine 125
exercise 264–6
after bypass surgery
after heart attack 151–4
and angina pain *79*, 80, 81, 136
choosing most suitable 272–9
clothing 278
combined with diet 249
ECG (exercise) 83–4

following angiogram 90
gradual build-up/warm-up 153,
    267, 270, *273*
how much to do 270
lack of *12*
MET (metabolic equivalent)
    267–9, *268*
possible dangers 152
with purpose 278–9
safety 271
stopping smoking 18, 21, 267
for stress 63
suitable types 150
to develop collaterals 115
'treadmill' test 83, 283*g*
types good for heart 266, *268*
eyes
blurred vision 45, 119
dryness *41*
with palpitations 183
ezetimibe (Ezetrol) 60

fainting 201–2
family discussion 163
family history *see* heredity
fatigue *see* tiredness
fats (lipids) 11, 48, 48–9, 54, 73,
    226–36
in 100 g-portions *245*
cutting down intake 231, 259
high/low levels 230
polyunsaturates/monounsat-
    urates 227, 284*g*, 286*g*
reduced fat products 234
saturated/unsaturated 50–1, 55,
    226–7, 286*g*, 287*g*
trans fatty acids 51, 283*g*
types 50–1
see also cholesterol; diet

felodipine (Plendil) *38*, 42, *92*, 99,
    220
fenofibrate (Lipantil) *58*
fibrates 58, *58*
fibre 236–9, *236*, *245*
fibrillation *see* atrial fibrillation;
    ventricular fibrillation
fibrinogen 15, 283*g*
first aid *see* **emergencies**
fish 227–9, *227*, *232–3*, 243
flecainide 188, 189, 193
Flora Pro-activ 234
flour 238
fluid retention 160–1, 162, 169,
    174, 242
flushing *41*, 95, 99
fluttering sensation of heart 283*g*
    see also atrial fibrillation
fluvastatin (Lescol) *58*
flying *see* travel after surgery
food *see* diet; *main individual*
    foods, e.g. fish; meat
fosinopril (Staril) *38*, *168*
free radicals 51–2, 283*g*
fruit 18, 41, 52, 184, 237, 238, 260–1
potassium source 243
sodium levels *241*
frusemide *168*, 169, 174
gallbladder problems 78
gardening 122
garlic 127–8, 246
gemfibrozil (Lopid) *58*
gender
and angina 90
coronary heart disease 67–8
and risk factors *12*
and smoking 16
Syndrome X 90
work after heart attack 143

general practitioner (GP) 80
　angina medication 101–2
　angina tests 81
　emergency 136
　palpitations 182, 185
genes *see* heredity
gingko warning 130
ginseng warning 130
glucose *see* blood sugar levels
glyceryl trinitrate (GTN tablets or
　　spray) (Carvedilol Eucardic)
　　79, 92
　in heart attack 137
Gopten (trandolapril) *39*
gout 40, *41*
GP *see* general practitioner
grafts *see* bypass surgery
grains *236*
grapefruit juice problem 184
GTN *see* glyceryl trinitrate
gum soreness 42

haemorrhage, cerebral 282*g*,
　　283*g*
hair growth 43–4
halitosis 95
HDL (high density lipoprotein)
　　49–51, 66, 73, 235, 284*g*
headache *41*, 42, 45, 95, 99, 101
　alcohol, with medication 103
　with nitrates 171–2
health foods 52–4
heart
　anatomy 2–7, *3, 87, 114, 116,
　　176*
　　see also individual areas,
　　　e.g. pericardium
　'electrics' (conduction system)
　　8–9, *9*, 282*g*

function 1–2, 7–9
size 175–6
transplant 174–7, *176*, 287*g*
what can go wrong 9–10
see also cardiac; cardio-;
　coronary heart disease;
　symptoms of heart
　problems; valves of heart
heart attack (myocardial
　infarction) 4, 12, 283*g*, 284*g*
　cause 133–4
　diagnostic tests 139
　different from angina 78–9, *79*
　emergency 135, 137–8
　essential information 141–2
　the event itself 137–42
　fear of recurrence 144–5
　minor *134*, 136–7
　recovery 142–5, 155–6
　reducing risk 26, 133
　sexual activity 213–14
　survival rate 150
　symptoms 134–7, *134*
　warning signs 135–6
heart beat/rate 4, 7, 8–9, 41
　in angina 75–6, 96, 97
　atrial fibrillation 170, 189–95
　bradycardia 196
　and bypass machine 113–14
　dangerous rhythm 200
　dangerous slowing down 42, 96
　'extra wire' 181
　heart block 196
　ideal measurement 152–3, 277,
　　278
　missed beats 179–80, 183, 187–8
　St John's wort warning 130
　sexual activity 212–13
　sinus rhythm 191

taking pulse in exercise 274–6, *276*
in ventricular fibrillation 138
see also electrocardiogram; pacemakers; palpitations
heart block 196, 284*g*
heart disease *see* coronary heart disease; valves of heart
heart failure 4, 12, 157, 284*g*
  ACE inhibitors 171
  atrial fibrillation 191
  causes 158, 159–60, 163, 167, 205
  lifestyle problems 161–2
  medication 169–74
  symptoms 160–3
  tests 163–7
  treatment 167–9
Heart Protection Study 52
heart rhythm *see* heart beat/rate
heart-lung machine 114–15, 206, 282*g*, 284*g*
heparin 105, 194
herbalism 126–8
heredity 9–10, 12–13, 68, 284*g*
  cholesterol 54
  smoking risk 13, 68
heroin 67
hibernating myocardium 162–3, 167, 284*g*
high density lipoprotein (HDL) *see* cholesterol, high density lipoprotein
HOCM (hypertrophic obstructive cardiomyopathy) 159
'hole in the heart' *see* atrial septal defect (ASD)
holidays 123–4
Holter monitor *see* electrocardiogram (ECG), mobile recorder

home care 121, 138–9
homeopathy 126
hormone replacement therapy (HRT) 68–74
  advice clarified 73–4
  available therapy 71
  breast cancer 69–70
  contraceptive pill 69
  side effects 70–1
hospital treatment
  angiogram 85–91
  angioplasty 104–5, 139
  bypass surgery 113–19, 121, 125
  cardiac rehabilitation 152–3
  cardioversion 194
  Coronary Care Unit 138, 139, 140–1
  EPS test 187
  heart attack procedure 139–42
  insertion of pacemaker 197
  thrombolysis 139
  see also home care
HRT *see* hormone replacement therapy
Hydrenox/Hydrosaluric (hydrochlorothiazde) *38*, 40
hydrochlorothiazide combinations *39*
hydrochlorothiazide (Hydrenox, Hydrosaluric) *38*, 40
hydrogenation 51
Hygroton (chlorthalidone) *38*, 40
hypercholesterolaemia 48, 50, 61, 284*g*
hyperlipidaemia 284*g*
hypertension (primary/ secondary) 284*g*
  see also blood pressure, raised/high

hypertrophy of heart muscle 9, 158
hypnosis 20–1
hypoglycaemia 42, 65
hypotension 284*g*
    see also blood pressure,
    lowering of
Hypovase (prazosin) *39*, 43
hypoxia 284*g*
    see also oxygen
hysterectomy 70
Hytrin (terazosin) *39*

ICU *see* intensive care unit
Ikorel (nicorandil) *92*, 101, 219
Imdur (isosorbide mononitrate)
    92, 95, 98
immunosuppressive drugs 284*g*
    see also drugs, suppressing new
    heart rejection
impotence *see* erectile
    dysfunction
incompetence (leaking) of heart
    valves 204, 284*g*
indapamide (Natrilix) *38*
Inderal (propranolol) *38*
Inderetic (propranolol + bendro-
    fluazide) *39*
indigestion 76, 78, 92
    prolonged 135
indoramin (Baratol) *39*
infection and valve surgery
    209–10
inferior vena cava 5
inhalators, nicotine replacement
    23
Innovace (enalapril) *39*, 42
INR (International Normalized
    Ratio) 172
insertion sheath 105

insulin 65–6
insurance 112, 123, 198
intensive care unit (ICU) 118
International Normalized Ratio
    see INR
ions 98
irbesartan (Aprovel) *39*, 131, *168*
irbesartan + hydrochlorothiazide
    (Co Aprovel) *39*
irritability 135, 146, 147
ischaemia 284*g*, 285*g*
Ismo (isosorbide mononitrate) *92*
isosorbide dinitrate *168*
isosorbide mononitrate (Elantan,
    Imdur, Ismo, Monit, Mono-
    Cedocard) *92*, 95, *168*
isradipine (Prescal) *38*
Istin (amlodipine) *38*, 42, *92*, 99,
    220

jaw pain 76, *134*, 135
jobs *see* work
joules and calories 245

keloid (scar) 121, 284*g*
keyhole surgery 114, 120, 130
kidneys 1, 5, 29, 32, 42–3
    in heart failure 164, 170
    palpitation treatment 188

labetalol (Trandate) *38*
lacidipine (Motens) *38*
laser surgery 130
LDL (low density lipoprotein)
    49–50, 51–2, 56, 66, 73, 284*g*
legs
    clotting risk 72
    feeling of heaviness *41*, 96
    leg pain 32

swelling 42, 119
Lescol (fluvastatin) 58
lethargy see tiredness
Levitra (sildenafil) 220
libido 217
lifestyle 155–6, 175, 188, 249
Lipantil (fenofibrate) 58
lipids see fats
Lipitor (atorvastatin) 58
lipoprotein see cholesterol
Lipostat (pravastatin) 58
lisinopril (Carace, Zestril) 38, 42,
    140, 168
lisinopril + hydrochlorothiazide
    (Zestoretic) 39
liver 1, 57, 59, 164
longevity 56
Lopid (gemfibrozil) 58
Lopresor (metoprolol) 38, 41, 92
losartan (Cozaar) 39, 42, 131, 168
losartan + hydrochlorothiazide
    (Cozaar-Comp) 39
lungs 1, 78, 139, 160–1
    problems with amiodarone 189

Ma huang (Ephedra) therapy 130
magnetic resonance imaging
    see MRI
mammary arteries 113, 114
margarine 234
marijuana see cannabis
meat 231, 232–3, 241, 243, 259
media hype 43
medication
    with alcohol 103
    for angina 101–3
    atrial fibrillation 192–3
    cardiac ablation as alternative
        195

clot buster drugs 139, 148
combining medicines 173
danger of stopping one's own
    97, 102, 112, 148, 162, 218
forgetting to take tablets 102
grapefruit juice problem 184
heart attack 139–40, 141–2,
    147–8
heart failure 169–74
palpitations 183, 188–9
valvular heart disease 206
warfarin 87–8
see also drugs; individual
    drugs; treatment
meditation 20
memory loss 45, 97, 102
menopause and cholesterol 50
mercury 35–6
metabolic agents 103
metabolism of medications 184
methyldopa (Aldomet) 41, 44
metoprolol (Betaloc, Lopresor)
    38, 41, 92, 140, 168
mexiletene 189
mibefradil (Posicor) 38
Micardis (telmisartan) 39
micturition see urine
Million Women Study 69
Minoxidil 43–4
mitral valve 5, 6, 6, 175, 204
    atrial fibrillation 190, 192
    prolapse 284g
    prolapse (MVP) 204, 284g
    valvuloplasty 208–9
Modalim (ciprofibrate) 58
Moduretic 41
moexipril (Perdix) 39
money, saved through stopping
    smoking 18

Monit/Monit SR (isosorbide mononitrate) *92*, 95
Mono-Cedocard (isosorbide mononitrate) *92*
Monocor (bisoprolol) *38*, 41, *92*
monosodium glutamate 243
morphine 67, 139
mortality rate *see* death
Motens (lacidipine) *38*
mouth dryness *41*
moxonidine (Physiotens) *41*, 44
MRI (magnetic resonance imaging) scan 110, 198
murmurs, heart 164, 205–6, 285*g*
muscles
  heart 2, 5, *6*, 9, 10
  pain *58*
  tone and calcium supply 98
  see also cardiomyopathy; heart failure
myocardial infarction 284*g*, 285*g*
  see also heart attack
myocardium 28*g*, 162–3

nadolol (Corgard) *92*
narrowing of arteries *see* arteries, narrowing/blocking
nasal spray, nicotine replacement 23
Natrilix (indapamide) *38*
nausea 78, 135, 188
nebivolol (Nebilet) *38*
neck pain 76
necrosis 285*g*
negative feedback mechanism 65
nevibolol 219
Niaspan (nicotinic acid) 235
nicardipine (Cardene SR) *38*, *92*
nicorandil (Ikoral) 90, *92*, 101, 219

nicotine 14–15
  cost of replacement preparations 24
  gum 22–3
  nasal sprays/inhalators/tablets 23–4
  patches 22, 23–4
  side effects 23–4
nicotinic acid 235
nifedipine (Adalat, Adalat LA, Cardilate MR, Coracten XL) *38*, 42, 43, *92*, 99
nifedipine + atenolol (Tenif, Beta-Adalat) *39*
nisoldipine (Syscor MR) *38*, *92*
nitrates 78, 80, 90, *92*, 93
  with beta-blockers 98, 99
  with calcium antagonists 99
  heart failure *168*, 171–2
  how they work 93
  patches 95
  sublingual 94, 214, 216
  tablets to swallow 94–5
  with Viagra 219, 220
  see also glyceryl trinitrate (GTN)
nuclear magnetic resonance (MNR) 285*g* *see* MRI; nuclear (thallium) scan
nuclear (thallium) scan 163, 166, 167, 287*g*
nurses, specialist 138, 143
nuts 235, 238

obesity *see* weight
Odrik (trandolapril) *39*
oedema 160–1, 285*g*
oesophagus 165
oestrogen 68, 70, 71

'off-pump' in bypass surgery 114–15

oils (in food) 50–1, 227–8

open heart surgery *see* bypass surgery

orlistat (Xenical) 251

osteoporosis 69, 72, 73, 74

oxprenolol (Trasicor) *92*

oxygen 1, 2, 5, *6*, 7
  in angina attack 78, 97
  effect of nicotine 14–15
  and exercise 154
  in heart attack 133

pacemakers 124, 177, 187, 196–9, *199*, 285*g*
  batteries 198
  possible problems 198–9
  returning to activity 198
  temporary/permanent types 196–7
  what is involved 197

pain
  see chest/heart pain; leg pain etc.

painkillers 119

palpitations (arrhythmia) 10, 42, 75, 95, 127, 178–9, 285*g*
  blackouts 201–2
  coffee (caffeine) 246
  medication 188–9
  possible causes 182–3, 246
  in pregnancy 181
  self-help 182–6
  tests 185–7
  treatment 187–9
  types 179–81, 196–200
  see also atrial fibrillation; cardiac ablation; cardio-

version; heart beat/rate; pacemakers

paracetamol 119

PCI (percutaneous coronary intervention) 112

PDE5 *see* phosphodiesterase-5

Perdix (moexipril) *39*

pericardial effusion 10

pericarditis 10, 285*g*

pericardium (pericardial sac) 10, 285*g*

perindopril (Coversyl) *39*, 131, 140, *168*

perindopril + indapamide (Coversyl Plus) *39*

personality and stress 64

perspiration 42

PET (positron emission tomography) 163, 167, 286*g*

pharmacist advice 102

phosphodiesterase-5 (PDE5) 220

Physiotens (moxonidine) 44

physiotherapy 118, 153

phytotherapy 127

pindolol (Visken) *38*, *92*

pins and needles *41*

pipe smoking *see* smoking, pipe-smoking

placebos 52, 126, 219

plant therapy *see* phytotherapy

plaque 12, 56, 127, 285*g*

Plavix (clopdogrel) 88, 92

Plendil (felodipine) *38*, 42, *92*, 99, 220

pollution, car exhaust 133–4

Posicor (mibefradil) *38*

'pot' *see* cannabis

potassium 40–1, 170, 171, 184–5, 242

potassium channel activators *92*,
101
potassium-saving diuretics *38*,
40–1
pravastatin (Lipostat) *58*
prazosin (Hypovase) *39*, 43
pregnancy 181
Prescal (isradipine) *38*
prevention 13
progesterone 70, 71
propafenone 189, 193
prophylaxis, antibiotic 209, 286*g*
propranolol (Inderal, Beta-
Prograne) *38*, *92*, 97, 140
propranolol + bendrofluazide
(Inderetic) *39*
prostate problems 43
protein, and cholesterol 49
proteins 245
PTCA (percutaneous
transluminal coronary
angioplasty) *see* angioplasty
pulmonary artery *176*, 286*g*
pulmonary valve 5, *6*, 7, 286*g*
pulse 7, 274–6, *276*
pulse vegetables 237, 238

Questran (cholestyramine) *58*
quinapril (Accupro) *39*, *168*
quinidine 193

race
    calcium antagonists 42
    insulin resistance problem 66
    as risk factor 13, 14, 33, 37, 257
radial artery 104, 105, 113
raloxifene 70
ramipril (Tritace) *39*, 131, 140,
    168

ranolozine 103
rashes of skin *41*, 111, 189
rebound effect (blood pressure)
45, 148
recovery after heart attack 142–5
rehabilitation
    after heart attack 141–5, 146,
    151
    after surgery 122–3
rejection of new heart 175
relaxation 20, 62, 127
    before surgery 105
    and exercise 154
research, raloxifene 70
resins as medication 58
restlessness 119
rheumatic fever 204
risk factors 12–13, 33, 61–7, 286*g*
rosuvastatin (Crestor) *58*
roughage *see* fibre

'saggy bag heart' (thin muscle)
158
St John's wort warning 130
salt 37, 40, 169, 240–3, *241–2*
saphenous vein graft *114*
scan *see* nuclear (thallium) scan;
    PET; SPECT
scarring *see* keloid (scar)
Sectral (acebutolol) *38*, *92*
Securon (verapamil) *38*, 42, *92*,
    99
Selective Estrogen Receptor
    Modulators (SERMS) 70
self-help 34, 36–7, 63
    after heart attack 142–4, 150–6,
    169
    angina 91
    heart failure 174

palpitations 182–5
septum of heart 6, 7
SERMS *see* Selective Estrogen
    Receptor Modulators
sex problems 45–6, 211–12
    after heart attack 145
    after surgery 122, 214, 224
    beta-blockers 96
    blood pressure treatment 45–6
    casual sex 213, 215
    and heart failure 162
    K-Y jelly 223
    libido 217
    loss of interest 215–17
    posture 215, 216
    preparing after heart attack
        222–3
    Viagra 214, 218–21
    in women 222
    see also erectile dysfunction
        (ED)
shakiness and tremor 97
shock treatment
    see cardioversion
shortness of breath *see*
    breathlessness
sickness feeling *see* nausea
side effects
    ACE inhibitors 42–3, 171–2
    alpha-blockers 43
    amiodarone 189
    apomorphine (Uprima) 221
    beta-blockers 96–7
    blood pressure-lowering drugs
        41
    calcium antagonists 42, 99–100
    cholesterol-lowering drugs
        57–8, 58
    digoxin 188

drugs for palpitations 189
flecainide 189
herbal therapies 128–9
HRT 70–1
medications in general 45, 148
methyldopa (Aldomet) 44
moxonidine (Physiotens) 44
nicotine replacements 23–4
sex life 45–6
sildenafil (Levitra, Cialis) 220
simvastatin (Zocor) 58
sinus node 8, 9, 286g
sinus rhythm 191
sinus tachycardia 184
skin rashes 41, 111, 189
sleep problems
    after bypass surgery 119
    after heart attack 147
    nicotine replacements 23
    taking statins 58
    vivid dreams 96
smoking 4, 12, 16
    alternative therapies 20–1
    cessation clinics 26–7
    and cholesterol level 56
    cigars 17
    and contraceptive pill 69
    erection problems in men 136
    exercise effect 21
    filters 25
    herbal/dummy cigarettes 25
    meditation 20
    passive 13–14, 285g
    pipe-smoking 17
    quitting/stopping 16–17, 17
        advice 18–20
        before bypass surgery 118
        drugs 26
        reasons for stopping 18

withdrawal symptoms 22
reducing 15
risks involved 13–27, *16*, 26, 68
'safe' cigarettes 14–15
saving money 18
starting up again 20
support groups 25
weight problems 21
see also nicotine
snoring 135
sodium *241–2*, 242–3, 286*g*
see also salt
specialist *see* cardiologist
SPECT (single photon emission
computed tomography) 166,
167
sphygmomanometer 8, 35–6, *35*,
286*g*
spironolactone (Aldactone) *38*,
41, *168*, 174
sports and risk 159, 199
sputum 118, 160
starch *see* fibre
Staril (fosinopril) *38*
statins 57–8, *58*, 60, 65, 101
heart failure 173
to prevent recurrence of
angina/heart attack 131,
141, 155
statistics
angina incidence 75
angiogram procedure risk 88
angioplasty success 107, 111,
1112
beta-blockers and survival rate
148
bypass surgery success 116–17
clot buster drugs benefit 149
clotting in legs 72

coronary artery disease 132
coronary heart disease 1–2
death and smoking 14, 25
heart attack survival rate 150
heart failure incidence 157
heart transplant success 175
HRT 69–70
hypertrophic cardiomyopathy
incidence 159
lowering cholesterol levels 55–6
raised blood pressure 31–3, *32*
stent use 108, 109
survival after valve replacement
207–8
stenosis (narrowing) 104, 204,
286*g*
of heart valves 204
see also angioplasty; coronary
arteries, blocking/
narrowing
stent 105, 107, 123–4, 286*g*
drug-eluting type 109, 111
how it works 108
reasons for insertion 108–9,
109, 149
sternum *see* breast bone
steroids (anabolic) 266
stethoscope 35–6, *35*, 286*g*
stomach upsets *41*, 58, 78, 90, 172
streptokinase 149, 286*g*
stress *12*, 20, 31, 46
casual sex 213
causing pain 78
coronary heart disease 61–5
and exercise 154
and the heart 2
palpitations 179, 187–8
personality 64
reducing levels 62–3, 64–5, 127

stroke 32, 36–7, 149, 286*g*
subclavian vein 197, 200
suffocation sensation 161
sugar 239–40, 245
suicide thoughts 147
sunlight sensitivity 189
superior vena cava 5
surgery 130
  for angina 104–25
  for heart failure 174–7
  resuming sexual activity after-
    wards 214
  for valvular disease 206–9
  *see also individual operations
    and procedures*
sweating
  after bypass surgery 119
  with pain 78, 135
swimming 151
syncope 286*g see* fainting
Syndrome X 90–1
Syscor MR (nisoldipine) *38*, *92*
systole 7, 8, 286*g*

tablets
  forgetting to take 48, 102
  for raised blood pressure 44–7
  taken with cold remedies 102
tachycardia 181, 184, 287*g*
tadalafil (Cialis) 220
tamoxifen 70
tar in smoking 14, 17, 25
teeth 117, 209, 239
telmisartan (Micardis) *39*
Tenif (atenolol + nifedipine) *39*
Tenoret 50/Tenoretic (atenolol +
  chlorthalidone) *39*, 42
Tenoretic (atenolol + chlorthalidone) *39*, 42

Tenormin (atenolol) *38*, 41, *92*,
  140
terazosin (Hytrin) *39*
tests
  angina 81–91
  atrial fibrillation 192
  biopsy 175, 280*g*
  chemical tests for heart attack
    139, 140, 170
  heart failure 163–7
  lipid profile 48, 56–7, 73
  palpitations 185–7
  preparation for bypass surgery
    117
  raised blood pressure 29
  thinness of blood 172
  valvular heart disease 205–6
  see also individual tests,
    e.g. angiogram
thallium 163, 166
thiazides 170
throat pain *134*, 135
thrombolysis 149, 287*g*
thrombosis *see* clotting of blood
thyroid gland 160, 164, 181
  causing atrial fibrillation 191,
    192
thyrotoxicosis 160, 184
Tildiem (diltiazem) *38*, 42, *92*,
  99
timolol (Betim, Biocadren) *38*,
  92, 140
tiredness 10, *41*, 43, 45, 96
  after bypass surgery 118, 124
  heart failure 162
  warning of heart attack 135
tissue plasminogen activator
  (TPA) 149, 287*g*
tobacco *see* smoking

TOE/TEE (transoesophageal
    echocardiography) 165–6
tolerance to medication 95
Totamol (atenolol) *38*, *92*
TPA (tissue plasminogen
    activator) 149
Trandate (labtalol) *38*
trandolapril (Gopten, Odrik) *39*,
    168
transmyocardial laser revascular-
    ization 130
transoesophageal echocardio-
    graphy (TOE) 287*g*
transplantation of heart
    see under heart
Trasicor (oxprenolol) *92*
travel 123–4, 161–2
    with pacemaker 198
treadmill 83, *83*
treatment
    after heart attack 147–50
    altering one's own 45
    cholesterol-lowering 57–60, *58*
    danger of stopping one's own
        97
    heart failure 167–77
    palpitations 185–9
    raised blood pressure 40–8
    valvular heart disease 206–9
    when feeling well 46–7
    see also angioplasty; drugs;
        hospital treatment;
        medication; side effects
tremor and shakiness 97
triamterene (Dytac) *38*, 41
tricuspid valve 5, *6*
triglycerides 48–9, 58, 73, 287*g*
trimetazidine 103
Tritace (ramipril) *39*

troponin (trop positive/negative)
    139

ultrasound 164–5, 283*g*
Univer (verapamil) *38*, 42, *92*, 99
Uprima (apomorphine) 221
urea level in blood 170
urine frequency 45, 169–70,
    201–2

vagus nerve 183
valsartan (Diovan) *39*, 42, 131,
    168, 171
valves of heart 3, *3*, 5–7, *6*, 7
    artificial valves 207
    damage 9, 67, 167
    narrow or leaking valve 158,
        204, 205
    valve disease 203–4
        causes 204
        infection 209–10
        surgery 160, 206–9
        symptoms 205
        tests 205–6
        treatment 206–9
    see also angiogram, coronary;
        aortic valve; mitral valve;
        ventricles
vardenafil (Levitra) 220
Vascace (cilazapril) *38*
vegetables *232*, 238, 239, 260–1
veins 2–3, 5, 113, *114*, 187, 287*g*
    insertion of pacemaker 197
    see also individual names,
        e.g. cephalic vein; superior
        vena cava
ventricles
    angiogram procedure 87, 88,
        287*g*

right and left 5, *6*, 7, *176*, 190, *199*
ventricular fibrillation 138, 283*g*
ventricular tachycardia 181
ventricular septal defect (VSD) 7, 287*g*
verapamil (Securon, Cordilox, Univer) *38*, 42, *92*, 99
Viagra 214, 218–22
vision *see* eyes, blurred vision
Visken (pindolol) *92*
vitamins 51–2, 238–9, 287*g*
vomiting 135, 188
VSD *see* ventricular septal defect

walking 19
   after heart attack 150–1
   and angina 79, 80, 83–4
   as exercise 272–8, *273–5*
   pain in legs 32
warfarin 87–8, 90
   and amiodarone 189
   for atrial fibrillation 193, 194
   and gingko 130
   for heart failure 172, 173
   with mechanical heart valves 207
   and nicotine 23
water, drinking plenty 18
water retention 42, 44
water tablets *see* diuretics
weather affecting angina 80
weight
   Body Mass Index (BMI) 252–4
   high blood pressure risk *12*, 33

ideal 252–3
loss through exercise 154
maintaining 252
obesity and heart disease 61, 66, 154, 257, 285*g*
reduction through diet 37, 39, 55, 154, 249–63
   Atkins diet 256
   general tips 249–51
   Weight Watchers 256–7
and smoking 1
waist/hip ratio 254, *255*
wheezing *41*, 96, 160
wine *see* alcohol
women
   coronary heart disease 67–74
   menopause and cholesterol 50, 73
   Viagra 222
   see also gender
work
   after bypass surgery 124
   early retirement 143
   and stress 61–3

X-ray 39, 85, 121
   of chest in heart failure 163–4
Xenical (orlistat) 251

Zestoretic (lisinopril + hydro-chlorothiazide) *39*
Zestril (lisinopril) *39*, 42
Zocor (simvastatin) *58*
Zyban (buproprion) 26

The '*At Your Fingertips*' guide Feedback Form

We hope that you found this '*at your fingertips*' guide helpful. We always appreciate readers' opinions and would be grateful if you could take a few minutes to complete this form for us.

❶ How did you acquire your copy of this book?

From my local library □

Read an article in a newspaper/magazine □

Found it by chance □

Recommended by a friend □

Recommended by a patient organisation/charity □

Recommended by a doctor/nurse/advisor □

Saw an advertisement □

❷ How much of the book have you read?

All of it □

More than half of it □

Less than half of it □

❸ Which copies/chapters have been most helpful?

....

....

❹ Overall, how useful to you was this '*at your fingertips*' guide?

Extremely useful □

Very useful □

Useful □

❺ What did you find most helpful?

....

....

6 **What did you find least helpful?**

....

....

7 **Have you read any other health books?**

Yes ☐   No ☐

If yes, which subjects did they cover?

....

....

How did this *at your fingertips* guide compare?

Much better   ☐

Better   ☐

About the same   ☐

Not as good   ☐

8 **Would you recommend this book to a friend?**

Yes ☐   No ☐

Thank you for your help. Please send your completed form to:

Class Publishing, FREEPOST, London W6 7BR

Surname _____ First name _____

Title Prof/Dr/Mr/Mrs/Ms _____

Address _____

Town _____ Postcode _____ Country _____

☐ Please add my name and address to receive details of related books
   [*Please note, we will not pass on your details to any other company*]

(HEART HEALTH AYF 2004)

Have you found **Heart Health – the 'at your fingertips' guide** useful and practical? If so, you may be interested in other books from Class Publishing.

Stop that heart attack!
NEW THIRD EDITION TO BE
PUBLISHED JANUARY 2004
Dr Derrick Cutting   £14.99
This fully updated third edition of
Dr Cutting's manual shows us his easy,
drug free and medically accurate way to
cut your risk of suffering a heart attack
dramatically.

Diabetes – the 'at your fingertips' guide
FIFTH EDITION   £14.99
*Professor Peter Sönksen, Dr Charles Fox
and Sue Judd*
Over 460 questions on diabetes are
answered clearly and accurately – the
ideal reference book for everyone with
diabetes.
　　'I have no hesitation in commending
　　this book . . .' – *Sir Steve Redgrave,
　　Vice President, Diabetes UK*

Parkinson's – the 'at your fingertips' guide
SECOND EDITION   £14.99
*Dr Marie Oxtoby
and Professor Adrian Williams*
Full of practical help and advice for
people with Parkinson's disease and their
families. This book gives you the
information and the confidence to tackle
the challenges that PD presents.
　　'An unqualified success' – *Dr Andrew
　　Lees, Consultant Neurologist, The
　　National Hospital for Neurology &
　　Neurosurgery*

Dementia: Alzheimer's and other dementias – the 'at your fingertips' guide
SECOND EDITION   £14.99
*Harry Cayton, Dr Nori Graham and Dr
James Warner*
At last – a book that tells you everything
you need to know about Alzheimer's and
other dementias. An invaluable
contribution to understanding all forms of
dementia.

High Blood Pressure – the 'at your fingertips' guide
NEW THIRD EDITION   £14.99
*Dr Tom Fahey, Professor Deirdre Murphy
with Dr Julian Tudor Hart*
The authors use all their years of
experience as blood pressure experts to
answer your questions on high blood
pressure.
　　'Readable and comprehensive
　　information' – *Dr Sylvia McLaughlan,
　　Director General, The Stroke
　　Association*

Stroke – the 'at your fingertips' guide
*Dr Anthony Rudd, Penny Irwin
and Bridget Penhale*   £14.99
This essential guidebook tells you all
about strokes – most importantly how to
recover from them. As well as providing
clear explanations of the medical
processes, tests, and treatments, the
book is full of practical advice, including
recuperation plans; you will find it
inspiring.

Asthma – the 'at your fingertips' guide
THIRD EDITION   £14.99
*Dr Mark Levy, Professor Sean Hilton
and Greta Barnes*
This book shows you how to keep your
asthma – or your family's asthma – under
control, making it easier to live a full,
happy and healthy life.
　　'This book gives you the knowledge.
　　Don't limit yourself.' – *Adrian
　　Moorhouse MBE, Olympic Gold
　　Medallist*

Cancer – the 'at your fingertips' guide
THIRD EDITION   £14.99
Val Speechley and Maxine Rosenfield
This invaluable reference guide gives you
clear and practical information about
cancer. Whether you have cancer
yourself, or are caring for someone who
does, you will find in this book the
information you need to reassure
yourself, and enable you to take control.

PRIORITY ORDER FORM

Cut out or photocopy this form and send it (post free in the UK) to:
Class Publishing Priority Service
FREEPOST
London W6 7BR

Please send me urgently
(tick boxes below)

*Post included
price per copy (UK only)*

☐ **Heart Health – the 'at your fingertips' guide**
(ISBN 1 85959 097 7)   £17.99

☐ **Stop that heart attack!**
(ISBN 1 85959 096 9)   £17.99

☐ **High Blood Pressure – the 'at your fingertips' guide**
(ISBN 1 85959 090 X)   £17.99

☐ **Diabetes – the 'at your fingertips' guide**
(ISBN 1 85959 087 X)   £17.99

☐ **Stroke – the 'at your fingertips' guide**
(ISBN 1 872362 98 2)   £17.99

☐ **Parkinson's – the 'at your fingertips' guide**
(ISBN 1 872362 96 6)   £17.99

☐ **Asthma – the 'at your fingertips' guide**
(ISBN 1 85959 006 3)   £17.99

☐ **Dementia: Alzheimer's and other dementias – the 'at your**   £17.99
fingertips' guide (ISBN 1 85959 075 6)

☐ **Cancer – the 'at your fingertips' guide**   £17.99
(ISBN 1 85959 036 5)

TOTAL _____

Easy ways to pay

Cheque: I enclose a cheque payable to Class Publishing for £ _____

Credit card: Please debit my

☐ Mastercard   ☐ Visa   ☐ Amex   ☐ Switch

Number _____ Expiry date _____

Name _____

My address for delivery is _____

_____

Town _____ County _____ Postcode _____

Telephone number *(in case of query)* _____

Credit card billing address if different from above _____

_____

Town _____ County _____ Postcode _____

Class Publishing's guarantee: remember that if, for any reason, you are not satisfied with these books, we will refund all your money, without any questions asked. Prices and VAT rates may be altered for reasons beyond our control.

☐ Please send me details of other Class Publishing titles that may be of interest to me.